Good For What Ails You

Dayton's Golden Age of Patent Medicine
by
Curt Dalton

Also by Curt Dalton

A is for America
The breweries of Dayton: An illustrated history
Curt Dalton's Gem City Jewels
Dayton (Postcard History Series)
The Dayton Arcade: Crown jewel of the Gem City
The Dayton Canoe Club: An illustrated history 1913-1996
Dayton inventions: Fact and fiction
Delicious recipes and food for thought from the NCR Archive
Good for what ails you: Dayton's golden age of patent medicine
Greater Dayton drive-in theatres: An illustrated history
Home Sweet Home Front: Dayton During World War II
How Ohio helped invent the world: From the airplane to the yo-yo
Keeping the secret: The WAVES and NCR Dayton, Ohio 1943-1946
Miami Valley's marvelous motor cars
Mr. Wulff's eagle-powered balloon
Spilt blood: When murder walked the streets of Dayton
A taste of Frigidaire
The terrible resurrection
Trotwood-Madison Community Cookbook
Through flood, through fire
When Dayton Went to the Movies
With Malice Toward All: The Lethal Life of Dr. Oliver C. Haugh

All Rights Reserved

Copyright 2008 by Curt Dalton
3236 Wonderview Drive
Dayton, OH 45414
email: cdalton@woh.rr.com

Acknowledgments

This book would not have been possible without the help of a number of people, many of whom I have never met. When I put out the word that I wanted to write about the patent medicine industry of Dayton collectors from across the United States and even overseas contacted me to share their bottles, trading cards and other materials. Their generosity resulted in the book that you now hold in your hands.

My thanks to Mike Smith of Yucca Valley, California; Dana Wiehl, of Bridgewater, Connecticut; Marianne Foster, of Richmond, Indiana; James D. Julia, Inc., Auctioners, of Fairfield, Maine, John Bartley of North Hampton, Ohio; John "Digger" Odell, bottle collector and book writer extraordinaire, of Mason, Ohio; Friends of Hayner for the items located in the Hayner Distillery Exhibition, Troy-Hayner Cultural Center in Troy, Ohio; John McCutcheon, of Milton, Vermont; and Nick Blackburn, of London, England.

Locally I want to thank Scott and Carol Davis, Carole Medlar, Librarian at the Dayton Metro Library; Frank Miller, of Mill-Cliff Books; Larry Sizer, John Wolf, and especially Dave Musselman for his help and expertise of all things Dayton.

For those of you I have missed mentioning, and for those of you who have asked not to be mentioned, I thank you as well. I have spoken to some really wonderful people during the writing of this book and am reminded, yet again, of Dayton's influence on the world, both past and present.

I hope you enjoy this book as much as I did researching it.

Curt Dalton

Table of Contents

Acknowledgments 3
Table of Contents 4
Introduction 5
Patent Medicines - What were They? 7
The Lure of Patent Medicines 9

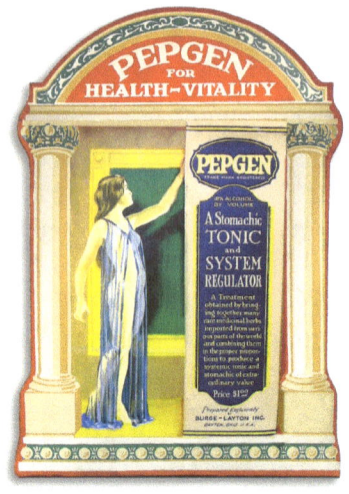

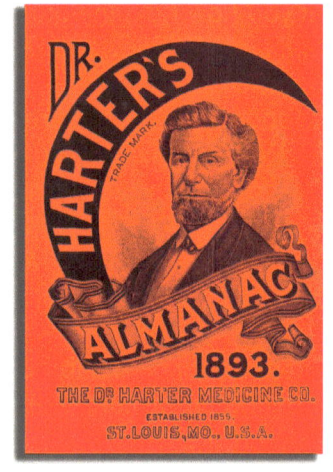

Cure-Alls 13
Doctors 18
Dr. Harter Medicine Company 24
Cooper Medicine Company 29
Druggists 36

Back to Nature 44
Indian Medicines 51
Miscellaneous Nostrums 55
Blackburn Products Company 64
Unmentionable Ailments 70

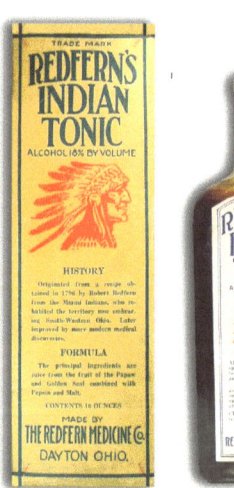

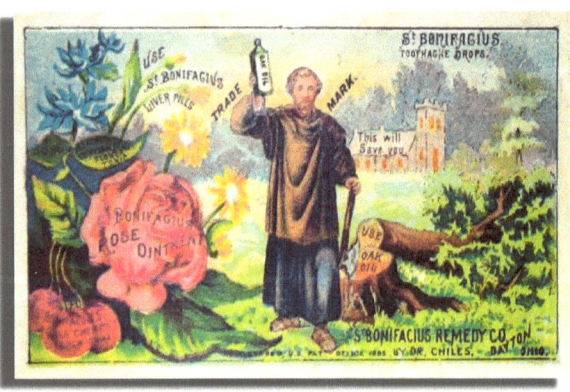

Vanity Nostrums 75
Testimonials 79
The Art of Advertising 84
The Decline of Patent Medicines 89
Patent Medicine Sellers 1850-1933 91
Index & Photo Credits 98

Introduction

Most times patent medicine salesmen and manufacturers are painted with a broad brush as charlatans who deliberately sold remedies they knew had no chance of working. Sometimes this wasn't the case at all, especially for the ones who made and sold remedies out of their homes. Many of the cure-alls involved recipes passed down from the previous generation. Personal experience convinced the seller and, in turn, their belief in the product sold their neighbors and friends. Think of someone who is certain that a particular vitamin helps them with their memory or diabetes or weight loss. Their belief leads others around them to believe as well, who in turn get the vitamins if they have the same problem. There is no fraud involved, just advice given by a well-meaning friend. Ministering to family and friends, many times these honest makers of home cures fulfilled a genuine need in their neighborhood.

Trouble is, as time passed, the cures were no longer in the hands of well-meaning people, but those of millionaire businessmen out to profit from other people's fear and suffering. While a home-healer relied on word-of-mouth, the larger patent medicine maker depended on newspapers, traveling medicine shows, almanacs and sometimes even fake testimonials to sell his merchandise. Many of these same nostrum makers knew that their products were useless, selling remedies that sometimes were more dangerous than the disease they were advertised to cure. That is why patent medicines and their makers have such a terrible reputation.

This book contains but a sampling of the potions, tonics, liniments and cure-alls manufactured in Dayton from around 1850 to the 1930s. In the back of the book is a list of well over 200 individuals and companies who advertised themselves as either making or selling patent medicines. Seventy-plus years after the fact, it is difficult to determine which medicine makers truly believed in their products and which remedies actually worked. I have tried to be as fair and impartial as the evidence allows. I leave it up to you, dear reader, to decide for yourself.

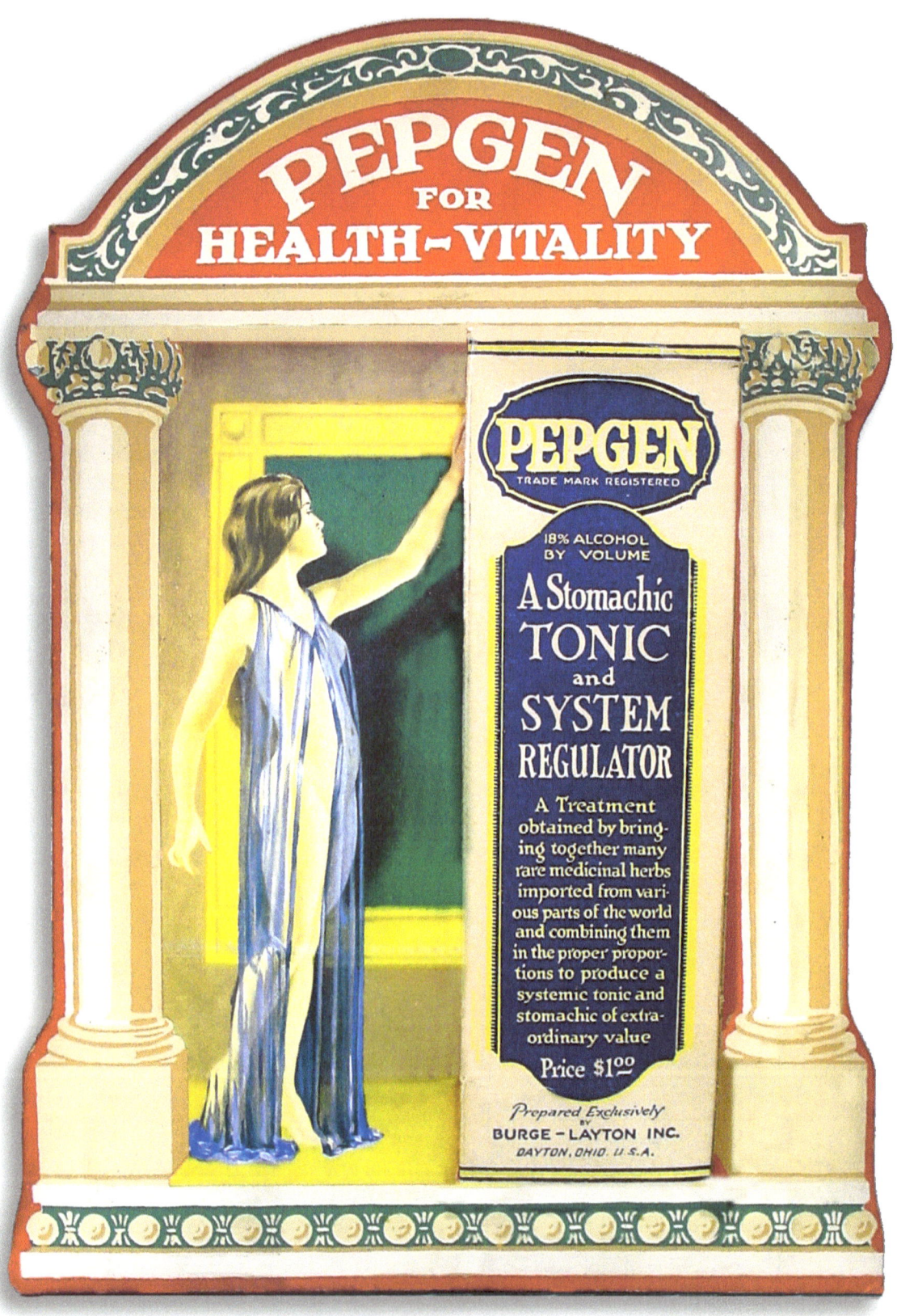

Many patent medicine manufactures spared no expense when it came to advertising. This eye-catching display used Greek architecture, vibrant colors, and a semi-clad woman to entice buyers to try Pepgen. The exotic setting enhanced the claim that the tonic was made of "rare medicinal herbs imported from various parts of the world." The tonic's 18% alcohol content was said to help preserve the herbs.

Chapter One
Patent Medicines - What Were They?

We all picture the pitchman from the old movies, pointing with his right hand at a bottle in his left, extolling the virtues of the "brown miracle in a bottle", a tonic that would cure your sore head, aching feet, depressed spirits or even any major diseases you may have.

The phrase "patent medicine" is deceiving in many ways. Rarely were the potions patented and most did not contain any curative ingredients. Then, as now, a patented invention did not need to work, but medicine makers were still leery of sharing their secret formulas, since the patent process would have required them to reveal the ingredients of their dubious products.

Some medicines really were patented, however. In 1863 Edward Conway, a dentist from Dayton, was awarded patent 37,901 for an "improved liniment." Called "Dr. E. Conway's Linimentum", the good doctor claimed his liniment could be used "for stopping of blood, the cure of rheumatism, cuts and inflammation of every kind." The amber colored transparent liniment was made up of brandy, camphor, cedar bark, hartshorn, ammonia, opium, orrisroot, white-oak bark and whiskey; ingredients sure to stop anyone's blood.

UNITED STATES PATENT OFFICE.

EDWARD CONWAY, OF DAYTON, OHIO.

IMPROVED LINIMENT.

Specification forming part of Letters Patent No. **37,901**, dated March 17, 1863.

To all whom it may concern:

Be it known that I, EDWARD CONWAY, of Dayton, Montgomery county, Ohio, have invented a new and useful liniment, called "Dr. E. Conway's Linimentum," for the stopping of blood, the cure of rheumatism, cuts, and inflammation of every kind; and I declare that the following is a full description of the same.

The nature of my invention consists in distilling, by any usual method, an amber-colored transparent liniment from the following described ingredients, used in the following proportions, by measure, and of the following strength, to wit: one part tincture of camphor, full strength; one part distilled hartshorn or ammonia, full strength; one part tincture of opium, full strength; one part extract of orrisroot, full strength, procured by distillation with spirits; one-half part extract of white-oak bark, procured by distillation with spirits; one-half part extract cedar bark, procured by distillation with spirits, the two last of full strength; one-half part fourth-proof brandy, and one-half part whisky, 35° above proof whisky. These ingredients, being all prepared separately, are mixed together, and from them is distilled, by any usual method, the liniment above described.

What I claim as my invention, and desire to secure by Letters Patent, is—

The production by distillation from the above-described ingredients, in the above-described amounts and strength, the above-described liniment for the stopping of blood, the cure of rheumatism, cuts, and inflammation of all kinds.

EDWARD CONWAY.

Witnesses:
JOHN HOWARD,
CHAS. PARROTT.

Dr. Conway's patent for "a new and useful liniment" was approved in 1863, making it a genuine "patent medicine". Eventually the term patent medicine was applied to any of this type of product, whether patented or not.

In many instances, even if the medicine itself wasn't patented, the owner made sure its trademark was. Most nostrums had colorful names, registered at the Patent Office, limiting the use of the name to the owner alone. Since the ingredients of the product weren't included in the register, the composition and use of the medicine could be changed at will, yet not effect ownership of the trademark.

Professionals in the field did not generally use the term "patent medicine", preferring the phrase "proprietary medicine". This implied that the product had been created by the owner, who also held the exclusive right to manufacture and sell the preparation.

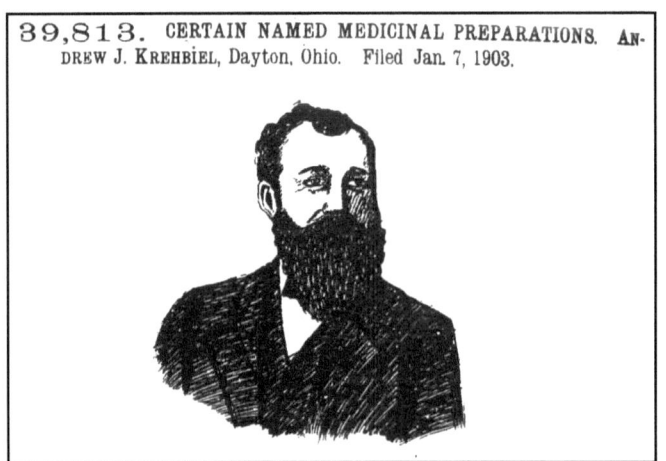
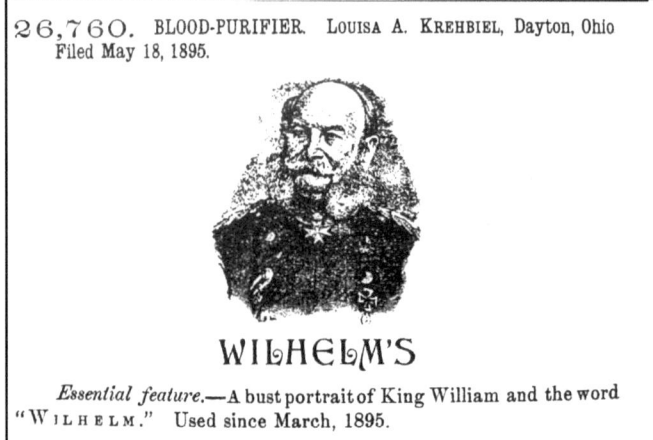

Examples of medicinal trademark patents granted to the Krehbiel family of Dayton at the turn of the century.

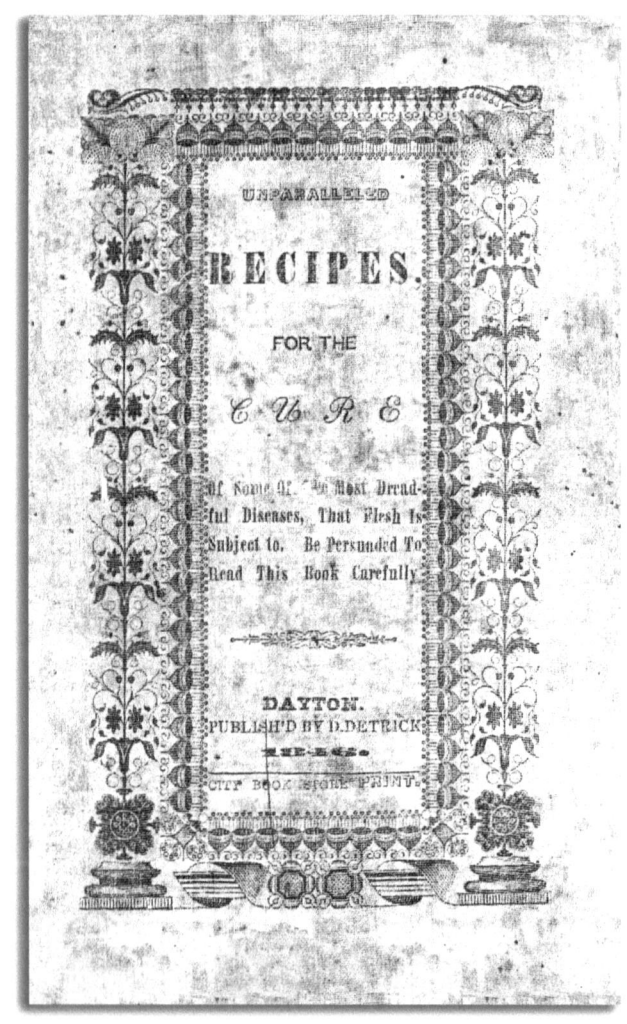

A popular item among many patent medicine sellers was the formulary, or "receipt" book. A sort of cookbook for druggists, these contained "recipes" for remedies that could be mixed, then sold in bottles labeled with their company's name. As we will see later, many patent medicine sellers skipped the recipes altogether, creating tonics, liniments and other concoctions with the cheapest ingredients possible, which had little or no medical benefits whatsoever.

There were also receipt books made for family use. In 1846, a book titled "Unparalleled Recipes for the CURE of Some of the Most Dreadful Diseases That Flesh is Subject to" was published by Daniel Detrick, of Dayton. It contained home remedies for ailments of all sorts, including fits, bleeding, cancer, burns and swelling. There was even a section in the back for cures of certain horse diseases. The book's recipe for the cure for cancer literally involved the use of toads and brimstone bubbling together in a kettle over a flaming pile of coal, bringing to mind witches mumbling "boil, boil, toil and trouble". It was no wonder that the good citizens of Dayton would reach for any other type of cure at all.

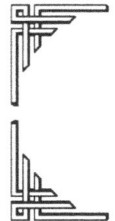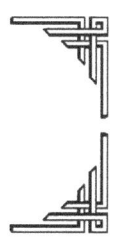

Chapter Two
The Lure of Patent Medicines

So what was the lure of these medicines? Doctors were few and far between and their knowledge of how the human body worked was limited at best. In fact, it wasn't until 1861 that the theory of germs was first published.

Terrible diseases raged in Ohio during the 19th century, and Dayton was no exception. In 1811 a sickness surfaced in Dayton that proved fatal to a number of children. At first the epidemic was attributed to "the sudden changes of this moist and variable climate," and parents were urged to guard their young against exposure. On December 9, 1811, the Centinel newspaper reported the funerals notices of four children who had died from the disease during the week, this at a time when the entire population of Dayton was less than four hundred people. It was later determined that it was the croup causing the fatalities. Before the era of immunizations and antibiotics, croup was a dreaded and deadly disease, which could cause the windpipe to swell shut. What was especially hard to bear was the fact that children under the age of 6 were usually the ones most affected. Although the croup eventually lessened its death grip on the children of the city, it never ceased to make a deadly appearance now and then over the years.

Dr. Job Haines was Mayor of Dayton in 1833 when cholera made an appearance in late June. Because of the grossly exaggerated reports which had spread through Ohio, Doctor Haines issued an official bulletin admitting an unusual prevalence of bowel troubles but denied the presence of cholera. Before the ink was dry with which the denial was penned, other cases occurred and established beyond question that cholera had reached Dayton.

People who contracted the disease began suffering from severe diarrhea, vomiting and cramps, some dying from dehydration in just a few hours after their symptoms first appeared. At that time, cholera patients were regularly prescribed calomel for their symptoms, a medicine containing mercury. Sometimes, patients who were fortunate to survive the disease in spite of the cure, suffered debilitating side-effects, or even died, from mercury poisoning. Out of a population of four thousand, there were thirty-three deaths between June and September.

In the fall of 1849, cholera again made its way through the city. The first fatal case of cholera was on May 18, 1849. It was discovered on a boat docked at the Dayton canal basin. Dr. M. Garst, who was in charge of the case, advised the authorities "to burn the boat and cremate the corpse." Had they followed his advice the epidemic in all probability would have been averted or greatly mitigated. But they did not.

The city must have sighed with relief as days passed and no one else died. Then, on June 13th, another fatality occurred, marking the beginning of a sixty-one day period of death and disease that lasted until mid-August. Business was almost entirely suspended until September, a Board of Health was appointed and a cholera hospital was established. The streets and alleys were white from the quantities of lime that was scattered in them.

In the end, the total deaths from cholera in Dayton that year came to two hundred and twenty-five, or one out of every forty-four people.

Drs. David S. Newman and Silas H. Smith were two dedicated physicians who cared for dozens of patients during the crisis. Unfortunately, both men succumbed to the disease, Dr. Smith dying on July 13th, followed three days later by Dr. Newman. Both were buried at Woodland. Though thought of as heroes, their deaths served as proof that even doctors didn't always know how to protect and cure themselves from diseases.

Many poorer Ohioans found doctors' fees to be exorbitant, ranging from fifty cents for an office visit to seventy-five dollars to remove kidney stones. Many patients paid their medical bills in produce due to their lack of cash. Unfortunately for both the patients and doctors, this practice precluded many physicians from buying more advanced medical equipment, further hampering medical care.

When a doctor was finally called upon, the

Fee Bill
adopted by the Montgomery County
Medical Society
May 29th 1851

Practice of Physic

For first visit in city		$1.00
" Subsequent visits to same case when once daily	each	.75
" Subsequent " to " " " twice or more daily	each	.50
" visits in Country first mile	each	$1.00
" visits in Country each additional mile (the second mile commencing at the Corporation line)		25¢ to 50¢
" Night visits 50 per cent additional charge may be added.		
" Detention with patient all night		$5.00
" Detention in day time	per hour	50¢
" May call		$1.00
" Consultation		$5.00
" Consultation subsequently in same case	each	$3.00
" Written Prescription		.50
" Written Opinion		$3.00
" Verbal Opinion or Advice		
" Prescription for each additional case in Family		50¢
" Opinion involving a question at law, in which a Physician may be Subpoenaed		$5.00
" Post Mortem examination in Cases of legal investigation		$10 to $20
" Certificate as Medical Examiner to Insurance Companies		$2.00

On May 29, 1851 the Montgomery County Medical Society Board adopted a list of fees for various medical procedures and practices. Amputation of a finger or toe ran upwards of five dollars, as did taking out each tonsil. Treating a patient for Syphilis cost up to $20 "to be paid in advance."

> *This little ditty was written about a Dayton doctor by the name of William Blodgett, who was running for a political office in the 1820's. Although it was published by his rivals, the meaning behind the poem is a fair indication of how people felt about all doctors in general at the time.*
>
> **As B- lay sick and 't was thought he was dying,**
> **His friends and relations around him were crying,**
> **Who made with their plaints such a terrible din,**
> **That Death who was passing and heard it went in.**
> **What the deuce, said the daemon, good folks, is the matter,**
> **That ye make around the doctor so devilish a clatter ;**
> **I'm not come to hurt him, so leave off your whining,**
> **You've no reason to tear me, altho' I look grim,**
> **For I know my own interest too well to kill him.**

patient sometimes had to endure nothing short of what would be considered torture today, in the hope of being cured of his ills.

The diary of Dr. Job Haines, for the years 1816 to 1820, is located at the Dayton Metro Library. In it, many subjects of medical interest are discussed, including the case of a Mr. Burgess.

On the 29th of August, 1816, Mr. Burgess began vomiting, it was supposed, from eating unripe plums. Draughts of warm water to promote vomiting were given, followed by potassium carbonate and laudanum (an alcoholic solution of opium). When the symptoms persisted, he was bled, a common practice thought to help the patient relieve himself of 'bad blood'. Mr. Burgess seemed to improve and the next day, after a precautionary bleeding, went to his home four and one-half miles away.

On the third day, Dr. Haines was recalled, diagnosed phrenitis (inflammation of the brain), and immediately drew sixteen to twenty ounces of blood. His patient was ordered to take a laxative, and place epispastics (a medicine that causes blisters) on the back of his neck. The same routine of bleeding, purging, blistering and sweating was repeated daily until September 14th, when the patient had a fainting fit. Mr. Burgess cut himself and bled out another ten to twelve ounces of blood before the doctor saw him.

> *When I arrived near sunset I took twelve to fourteen ounces more from the jugular, applied an epispastic to the forepart of the head, and gave a cathartic. By these means he was in a measure relieved of pain, but not entirely. The pulse being tense and the pain severe, I bled him again this morning (September 15th) to fourteen ounces... In my absence during the day the pain returned and the pulse became tense. I had left my lancet with him and directed him to bleed if necessary. Accordingly he had a vein opened twice and lost twelve to fourteen ounces each time, so that when I arrived in the evening the pulse was soft and pain very moderate. I concluded to stay all night. Was called up about three o'clock on account of return of fever and pain and bled again to twelve ounces. I left in the morning, but during my absence the pain returned and he lost by two bleedings sixteen ounces of blood.*

On the morning of the 18th, the pain and fever returned, and the patient cut himself and bled out yet another sixteen ounces of blood.

Though greatly debilitated, Mr. Burgess did fairly well for the next thirty-six hours, until a sudden attack of head pain was seen as a signal for the letting of more blood, and fourteen ounces at two bleedings were taken from the jugular.

The final entry made on September 26th reads:

> *Mr. B grows stronger, but is troubled with dyspepsia, to which he is constitutionally subject.*

This brought an end to Burgess' treatment. He has experienced twenty bleedings, with a net loss to the patient of about seventeen pints of blood.

A few weeks later the diary makes note:

Clear and pleasant. Sale at Widow Burgess'.

The combination of fear of diseases, the shortcomings of the knowledge doctors had to cure them, and the amount of money the doctors charged, helped lead to the success of the patent medicine industry. Add to this the fact that often the tonics actually seemed to be help, due to containing ingredients such as opium, cocaine and a healthy(?) dose of alcohol, all of which would certainly make you feel better, at least for a little while. The tonics were cheap and could be self-administered, an advantage at a time where the practice of medicine leaned more towards the word "practice".

This isn't to say that all patent medicines were bad. Kaolin, ipecac and quinine were among the ingredients used by some potions that actually did have medical worth. But the sad fact was, most of the nostrum sellers depended on their knowledge that most people who become ill will get better again, whether they take any medicine or not.

The real cruelty came when patent medicine users held so much faith in the product they were using that they sometimes didn't seek professional help until it was too late. Other times, some users became addicted to the alcohol, morphine or cocaine the remedies might contain. The tonic "Kurokol", which was manufactured by the Cooper Medicine Company in Dayton, was 8 percent alcohol and contained chloroform and cannabis. The front of the bottle had recommended doses for children as young as one year old. The medicine was to be taken once an hour for four hours. "Children take it readily" the company claimed.

So, who were the people doling out these patent medicines? According to the Western Sun newspaper of Vincennes, Ohio, it could be anyone. On July 6, 1826 the editor lamented that:

Any idle mechanic, not caring longer to drudge at day labor, by chance gets a dispensatory, or some old receipt book, and poring over it, or having it read to him…, he finds that mercury is good for the itch, and old ulsers; that opium will give ease; and that a glass of antimony will vomit.
Down goes the hammer, or saw, razor, awl, or shuttle - and away to work to make electuaries, tinctures, elixirs, pills, plasters and poultices…Nothing can equal the ignorance of such empires but the stupidity of these people who buy their unwholesome preparations.

But it wasn't just the backdoor, self-proclaimed remedy maker that provided quack medicines. Even so-called professionals also got into the act. In the next chapter we'll take a look at examples of both type of sellers.

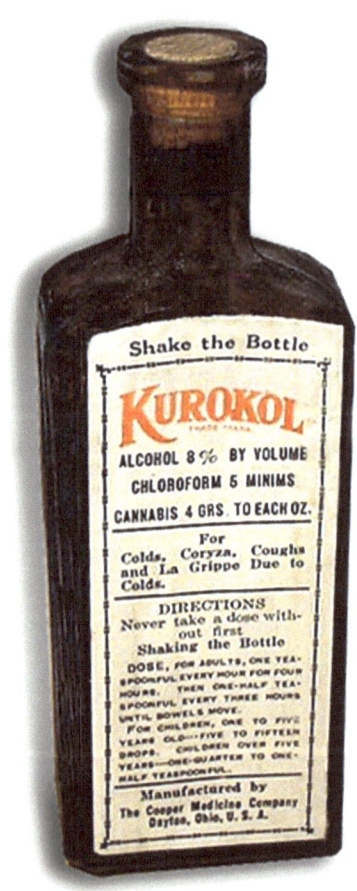

Made by the Cooper Medicine Company, Kurokol claimed to be good for colds, coughs, La Grippe and bronchitis due to colds, plus acted as a antipyretic, expectorant, laxative and an antiseptic. Each bottle came with a guarantee that if after four doses you weren't delighted, you could get your money back. With ingredients including alcohol, cannibus and chloroform, who wouldn't be happy, as well as fast asleep.

Chapter Three
Cure-Alls

Before the turn of the twentieth century, patent medicine manufacturers liberally used the word "cure" in their advertisements, some claiming that their product could cure almost every disease known to man, others promising to completely cure at least one ailment. This was especially true when it came to major diseases like cancer and tuberculosis. Unfortunately, while the "cures" themselves were usually not dangerous, many times a patient would rely on a worthless remedy until the disease had reached a point where it could no longer be treated.

How could the same people who were convinced that doctors knew nothing turn around and be persuaded that there was a cure for their condition after all? Much of this was due to desperation. Faced with a serious health problem that the doctors could not cure the sufferer would become desperate enough to try almost anything that would save his or her life.

Bowanee

The Bowanee Medicine Company was begun in 1889 by brothers Augustus and William Miller. Their product was also called Bowanee, which they advertised as "an unfailing cure for dyspepsia and all kinds of stomach troubles arising from indigestion." The two brothers soon sold their interests in the company to their bookkeeper Benjamin Green and his brother, Harry.

The Green brothers place a long ad in the form of a speech published by Bowanee in August 26, 1889 Sandusky Daily Register. "Bowanee first appeals to the people of Ohio, its native State. It makes no apology for the bold stand taken by it. It neither asks, nor will it give, quarter to those it deems guilty of deceiving and robbing the people. It enters the WORLD OF FRAUD, PATENT MEDICINE, with conquest inscribed upon its banner."

Bowanee's advertising approach was to claim that other patent companies were out to "deceive and rob poor sufferers (who) are not only fleeced of their money, but are sadly disappointed in their hopes." But, of course, the Bowanee Medicine Company was different. They promised "to give the people a BETTER MEDICINE" than had ever been offered before.

Bowanee admitted that no one medicine could cure everything and that anyone claiming that should be branded as frauds and cheats. Instead, Bowanee made broad claims that never really focused on all the diseases it could cure.

Bowanee's great mission is to cure a class of diseases all arising from the same cause, that are often met with the practicing physician and HARDEST TO CURE OF ALL AILMENTS afflicting the human race... THE STOMACH is the source and fountain of life, misery or happiness. Its diseases are the most stressing of all. Dyspepsia, Indigestion and diseases arising solely from these causes are the great common enemy of mankind. Bowanee comes nearer a SPECIFIC for these troubles than any medicine EVER TAKEN INTO THE HUMAN STOMACH. Upon this broad declaration will Bowanee stand or fall.

It didn't take long for the verdict to come in. The company had folded up its tent by 1896.

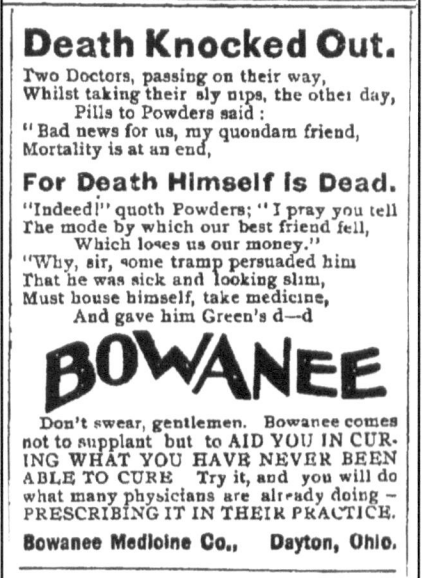

Dr. Livingston's Positive Cure for Catarrh

In 1888 E. B. Livingston and W. W. Hunter began the Dr. Livingston Medicine Company. Dr. Charles E. Livingston, of Dayton, was hired to be the company's business manager, no doubt in order for them to sell their product under the name of "Dr. Livingston's Positive Cure for Catarrh." The company caught the public's attention by placing ads in several newspapers across Ohio, offering a $1000 reward for "Every case of Nasal, Post Nasal, or Chronic Catarrh that Dr. Livingston's Positive Cure for Catarrh fails to cure." In smaller letters it explains that the reward is only good if "instructions and directions are carried out in FULL." The company also guaranteed that buyers would be relieved of their symptoms immediately, or their money would be refunded. It's a safe bet that anyone who wasn't happy with the product probably had a hard enough time getting the dollar back they paid for the bottle, let alone any chance of receiving the $1000 reward.

C. J. F. Daniels' Great Nova Scotia Pain Killer

C. J. F. Daniels was one of the many individuals who made and sold patent medicines from their homes. Starting in 1877, for fifty cents anyone could go to Daniels' home on Broadway in West Dayton and purchase a bottle of his "Great Nova Scotia Pain Killer". Daniels little bottle could cure nearly anything. Suffering from rheumatism, neuralgia, pains in the back or sides? Or perhaps a case of cholera, along with a sick headache and a sore throat? Chronic diarrhea or a case of piles? Daniels' nostrum did it all. And to top it off, it claimed it could even cure deafness.

There must have been some magic in that old bottle, for the company lasted for twenty-two years. When C. J. F. Daniels died in April of 1889, his wife Ann continued to sell the family potion until 1898.

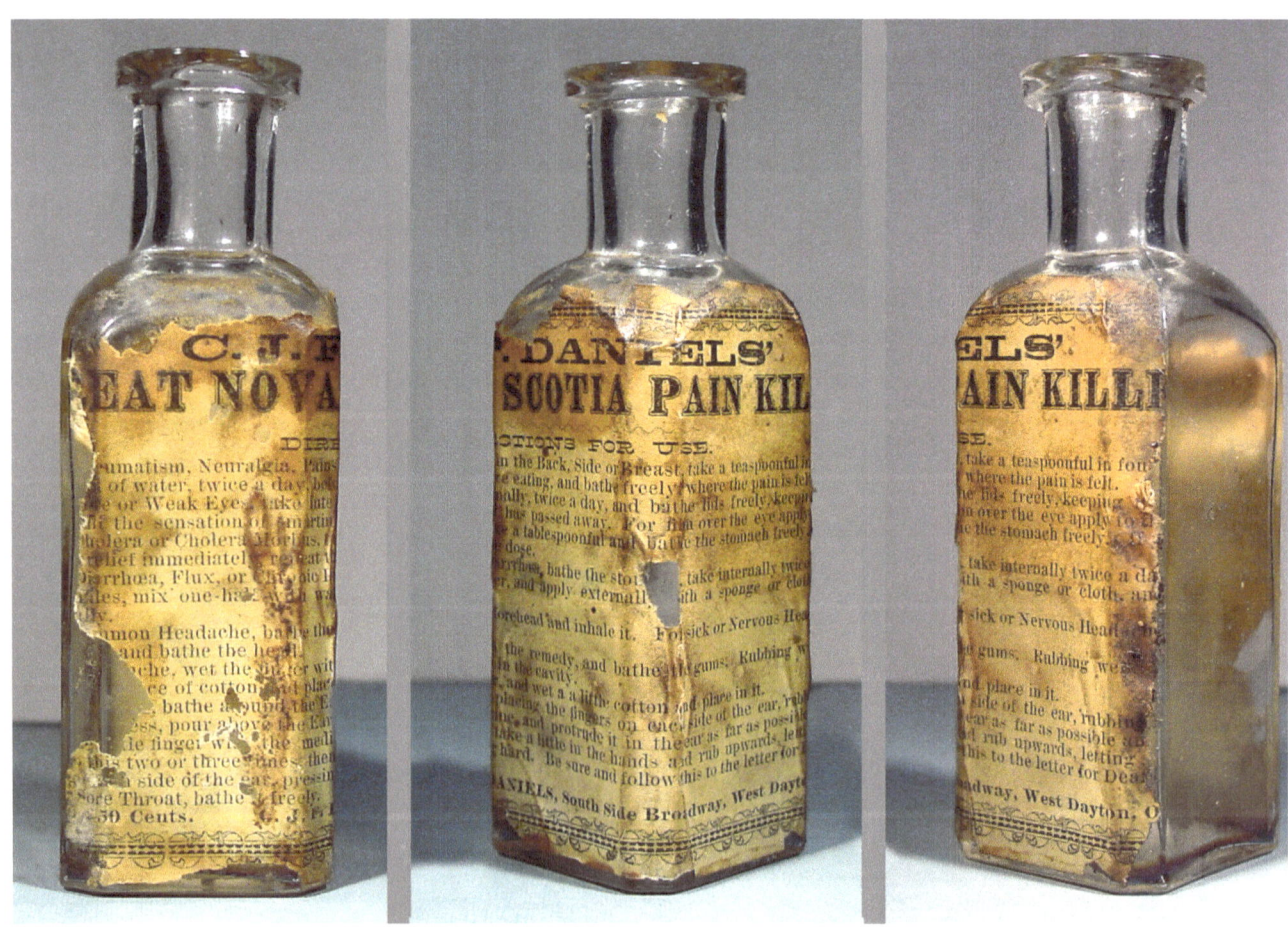

Rumex

While advertised mainly for constipation, Rumex was also suppose to cure "diseases of the Bone, Biliousness, Scrofula, Eczema, Tetter, Syphilis of any character, Rheumatism, Skin, Liver and Kidney Diseases". The Rumex Medicine Company advertised its medicine was guaranteed under the Food and Drugs Act of June 20, 1906 - a claim that might well have sold more product, but nevertheless was almost a toothless law at that point. The 1906 act focused mainly on prohibiting interstate commerce in misbranded and adulterated foods and drugs. As long as a company restricted sales to within its own state, it was staying within the boundaries of the law, no matter the promises made on its packaging.

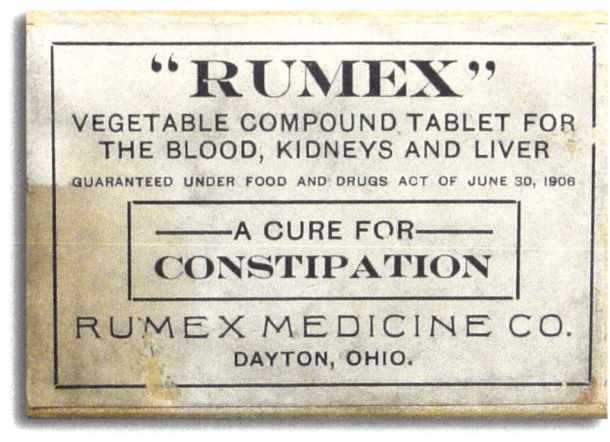

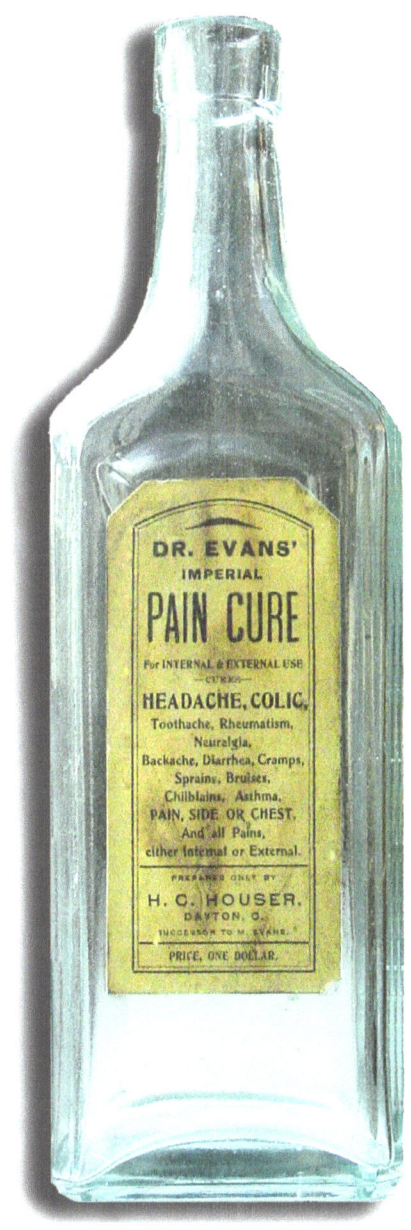

Dr. Evans' Imperial Pain Cure

Not much is known about this product or its manufacturers. The label seems to indicate that a Dr. M. Evans was the first to offer this nostrum which, besides curing an impressive list of diseases, also promised to end "all Pains, either Internal or External." It is not known whether Dr. Evans was from Dayton, but the bottle's label states that his successor, H. C. Houser, was. Users of Imperial Pain Cure were instructed to take one teaspoonful in warm water every half hour until relief was obtained. For external use, the medicine was to be rub in well with the palm of the hand. Every bottle came with a warrant of satisfaction if "used thoroughly."

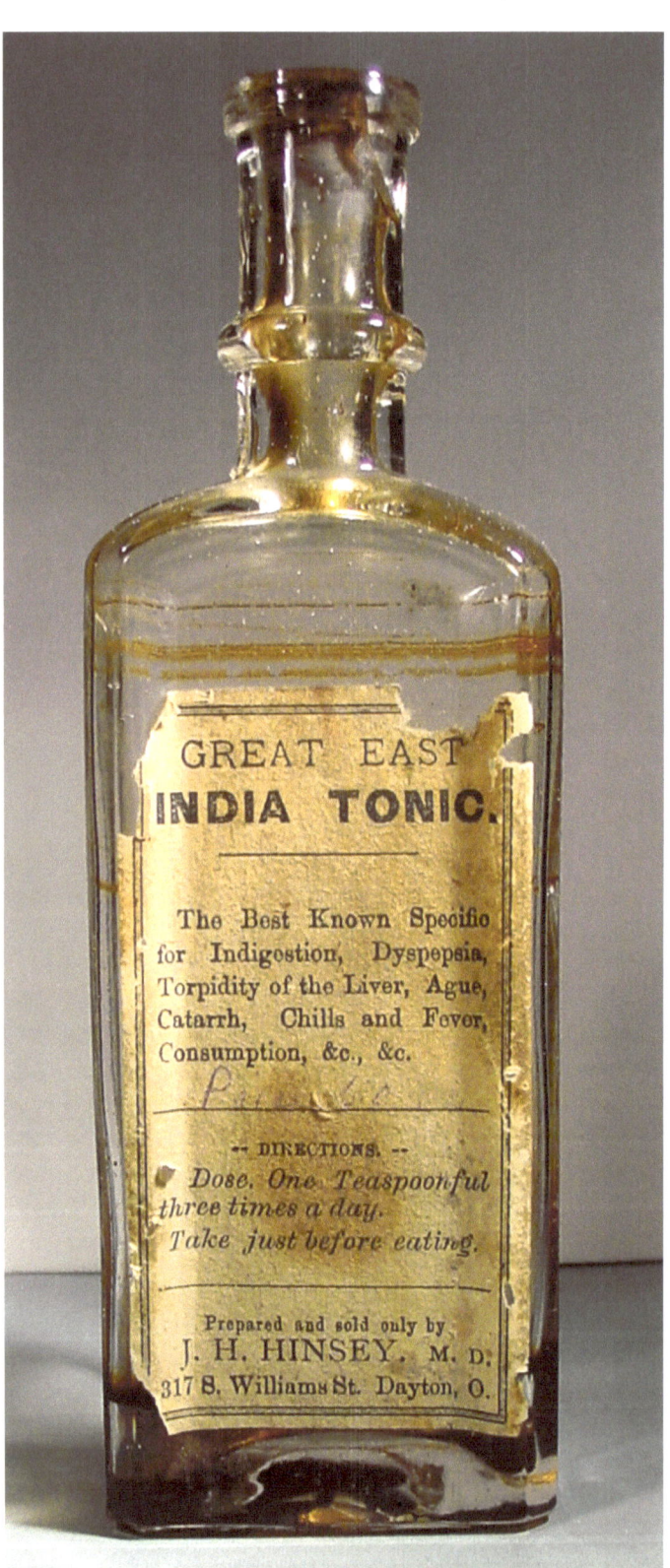

Great East India Tonic

In 1889 John H. Hinsey was working as a carpenter when, for reasons lost in time, he decided to get into the patent medicine business. He bought himself some bottles, had some labels printed and was soon selling "Great East India Tonic" from his home at 317 South Williams Street. A true salesman, Hinsey added the initials M.D. after his name, probably with the thought that this would lend legitimacy to his product. No records have been found by the author to indicate that "Dr." Hinsey ever received a medical degree.

Hinsey's miracle nostrum was advertised as the "best known" cure for several ills, ranging from indigestion to one of the most dreaded diseases at the time, consumption.

After John's death in 1906, his widow, Mary, would continue to sell the tonic until 1921.

The Gold Cure

In 1890, an unusual treatment by a real doctor was making the rounds, which was supposed to cure the effects of *other* cures. Many of the patent medicines of old contained alcohol and morphine and their users sometimes became dependent on their "medicine".

Dr. George H. Geiger, a well-known Dayton physician, claimed to have perfected a cure for alcoholism and morphine. According to the good doctor, men with drinking and drug problems had a disease that was produced by poisoning of the nerve cells. Fortunately, Dr. Geiger knew how to "cure" their problem. The remedy consisted of a strict dietary regime, accompanied by regular injections of 'bichloride of gold', a mixture of gold salts and vegetables. During the first few days, patients were allowed to consume as much alcohol as they wanted, provided that they allowed themselves to be injected four times a day with the "Gold Cure." Dr. Geiger claimed that patients who stuck it out for four weeks were cured over fifty percent of the time.

While it is not clear how successful Dr. Geiger's cure really was, at least for one patient it was an utter failure.

Bruno Kirves was a plasterer and very good at his trade. But during the lax winter months he was prone to drink more than usual. By 1898, Bruno was a confirmed alcoholic. A mean drunk, Kirves antics were worsened by the fact that he also suffered attacks of delirium tremens, or the DTs. Desperate to end his addiction, Kirves turned to Dr. Geiger for help. Regrettably, the gold injections didn't work. In order to lessen Kirves tremors and hallucinations, Dr. Geiger began prescribing a solution of chloral hydrate mixed in alcohol, also known as a 'Mickey Finn'. It wasn't long before Kirves became a slave to this habit as well.

Things came to a head on November 16, 1898. Bruno and his wife, Mary, began arguing. In his drunken state, Bruno threatened to kill her and their children. Mary yelled back that she was going to divorce him. This angered him to the point that he left the house and did not return home that evening.

About 9am the next morning Bruno made his way home, carrying a double-barreled shotgun. He entered the house through the back door and went to the living room where his daughter, Emma, was standing at the front door. As she started to turn, her father fired and Emma fell to the floor, dead. Kirves was soon captured and charged with her murder.

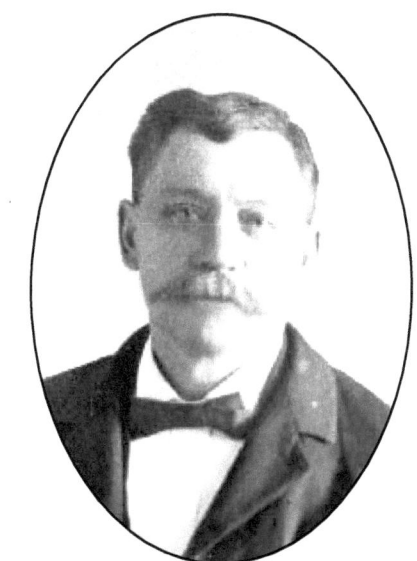

Bruno Kirves

During the trial a letter written by Dr. Geiger was entered as evidence. It read, in part:

I have been cognizant of the long continued intemperance of the said Bruno Kirves, and in my opinion, based on my experience in the treatment of inebriety, the said Bruno Kirves is unsound mentally...

Or, in other words, since the Gold Treatment failed to work, then Kirves *had* to be insane.

The jury believed otherwise and Bruno Kirves was executed for his crime on August 17, 1899.

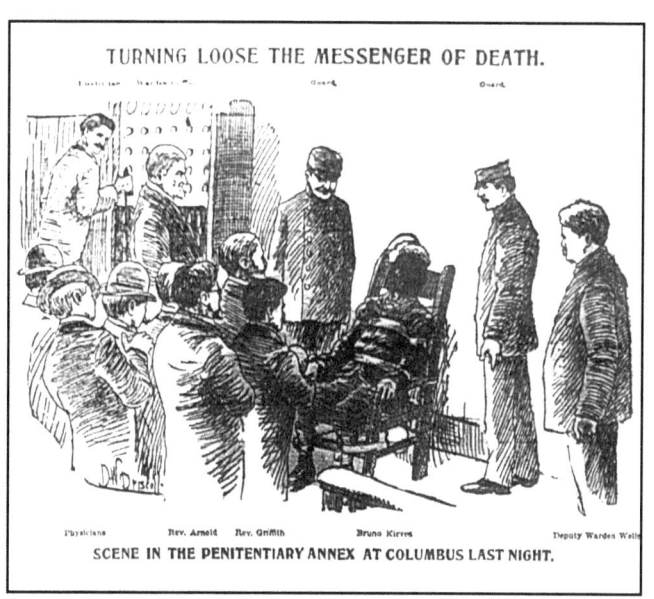

Chapter Four
Doctors

Local doctors soon found that people paid more readily for a bottle of medicine than a physician's fee. Yet doctors who turned to making their own remedies often had to bear the wrath of other physicians who believed that self-medication was not the proper way for people to take care of their health.

Dr. James S. Rose

If you wanted to pick out one of the strangest characters in Dayton's history, you wouldn't be far off the mark if you chose Dr James S. Rose. Dr. William J. Conklin once described Dr. Rose as "unquestionably the most unique specimen who ever masqueraded under the pseudonym, 'Doc'."

I can see him now leaning on his staff in the doorway of the old frame shanty on South Jefferson Street. Thin and wrinkled, and wizzen-faced, body bent to a quarter circle, eyes deep-set under shaggy brows, and small and piercing like a serpent's, beard, gray and long, covering the upper chest, a dressing-gown, red-figured and greasy, dangling from his misshapen shoulders, and an antique silk hat pushed far back over a bald and shining occiput - all in all, his appearance was uncanny enough to hurry school-children to their mothers' knees and to give rise to the story of a haunted house.

James S. Rose was born in North Marlboro, Massachusetts in 1817. After a stint as a clerk in a dry goods store there, James headed south and is thought to have worked his way through a medical college in Macon, Georgia. A love affair gone wrong sent Rose into a tailspin and he spent the next few years wandering the south. Much of this time was spent in the woods, and to the patients who sought his remedies after he began his practice, Rose would explain that he had concocted the medicine from herbs of his own discovery.

Dr. Rose finally drifted northward, landing in Dayton in 1857. Always dressed in a rather flamboyant suit and a black beaver hat, and considerably stooped over due to an injury to his spine as a boy, the good doctor made quite an impression on the city when he opened his office on Second Street between Main and Ludlow.

When he proclaimed to have discovered a cure of consumption the local doctors called him a quack. But they couldn't explain the fact that the pills and potions passed out by Rose actually did seem to work as well as, or better than, anything they gave their own patients.

By 1870 Dr. Rose had taken on a wife, as well as a desire to raise fancy chickens as pets. The hobby took on a life of its own, to the point that it finally became necessary for the doctor to find larger quarters, which he found in the form of an old dilapidated home on South Jefferson Street.

Completely spurned by the other doctors, Dr. Rose decided to show his contempt of the entire

Scrofula, also known as the "King's Evil", refers to tuberculosis of the neck. Dr. Rose ran this ad in the Dayton Daily Empire newspaper for several months, beginning October 22, 1860. In it, he claims to cure diseases that others cannot, something that was sure to have endeared him to local physicians

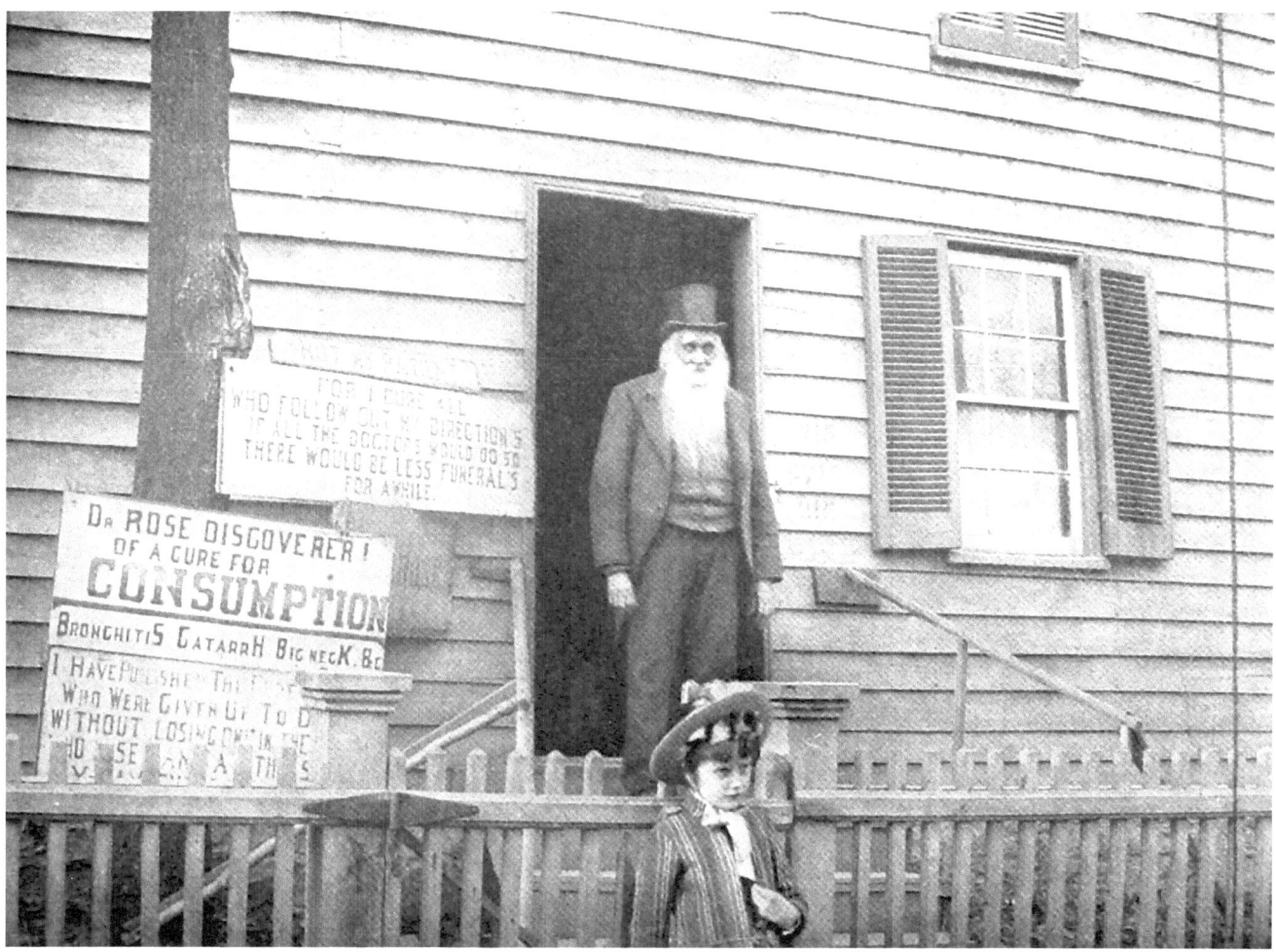

The grim humor of Dr. James S. Rose is best shown in the placards displayed on the outer wall of his shop. One read: "No poisoning or torturing, no burning and dissecting the living done here. Slaughter-pens farther up," referring to the offices of doctors on the same street.

medical profession by erecting a sign with gaudy lettering in front of his new home which stated:

**Dr. J. S. Rose Discoverer!
of a Cure for
CONSUMPTION
Bronchitis, Catarrh, Big Neck, etc.
For I Cure All
Who Follow Out My Direction's
If All the Doctors Would Do So
There Would Be Less Funeral's
For Awhile**

Underneath was hinged another, smaller board, which could be folded against the larger sign so as to hide the writing on it from view. Whenever a funeral procession would wind its way down Jefferson Street towards the cemetery, the eccentric old physician would step into the yard and drop down the little sign so that everyone could read its plain but powerful message:

NOT MY PATIENT

The sign caused an uproar of sorts. When the New York Tribune found out about the doctor's unusual marketing ploy, they mentioned it in a small blurb, with the heading "A Genius for Advertising". Soon the doctor found himself being mentioned in newspapers across the country.

Smelling a bigger story, a reporter decided to pay Dr. Rose a visit. After a long bout of questions through a narrow crack in the door, the doctor was finally persuaded to talk, but even then refused to reveal the secret formulas or name even one of the herbs he used in preparing his remedies.

Some of his views were quite modern.

Anyone can be cured of consumption if they want to be cured; the trouble is they don't want to," he stated. "I think that if people would leave tobacco and whiskey alone they wouldn't be so susceptible to this disease, and a lot of other diseases. Food you get nowadays is adulterated, so there isn't much that's fit to eat any more. For my part, I eat about one meal a day. I always rise at sunup and go to bed when I see my chickens going to roost. I've always made it a practice to eat when I was hungry. This thing of having regular mealtimes is foolish. We eat too often when we don't need it or enjoy it.

On May 26, 1894 Dr. Rose passed away. He had been ill for some weeks, but had refused to allow any of the local physicians to look in on him. His wife having passed away some eight years before, the doctor's only companion was a young boy who ran errands for him. As he lay dying, Dr. Rose continually called out for Augusta. Augusta Lannon was the name of the southern belle from Macon, Georgia who had broken his heart some fifty years before.

When the police came to get his body, they were greeted by an unusual sight. In the front room were hundreds of full and half-full bottles, large and small, stacked everywhere on shelves, chairs and tables. An old tin bucket stood to one side, filled with a quart of pills. In the brick building behind the house that Dr. Rose used as a laboratory, were found a wagonload of bottles and jugs, while on a bench along one wall rested a dozen wine casks which were filled with what the doctor had marketed as his favorite self-made remedy - "Strong Wine of Life." The fluid was dark brown in color and, as the reporter described it at the time, "ran like molasses on a summer day." In this room too, stood a number of tubs, boxes and barrels, all containing bottles of every size and shape.

Dr. Rose was buried at Greencastle cemetery. Ever unusual, even to the end, at the doctor's request a unique grave marker was placed at the head of the grave. It consisted of a polished board, one that had apparently served at some time as a supporting piece for a stair banister. It is unknown if Dr. Rose's name was carved into it.

Dr. Oliver Crook

Dr. Oliver Crook enjoyed the distinction of being the first native-born Montgomery County boy to enter the medical field. Born in Wayne township on August 14, 1818, he spent his boyhood working on the farm. After graduating from the University of New York in 1847, he opened an office in Dayton. After being in practice for several years, Dr. Crook went to the Eye and Ear Infirmary in New York. When he returned, Dr. Crook made these organs one of his specialties. He had partnerships with his brother-in-law, Dr. Koogler, then with his brother Dr. James Crook. James died in 1855. From that time until he began making patent medicines, Oliver was in practice alone.

Curiously, Dr. Crook's troubles began from associating with a Dr. Geiger. Not the one of Gold Cure fame, however. In October 1857 Dr. Oliver Crook was taken to task by the Montgomery County Medical Society for consulting with a Dr. Alburtus Geiger, "a man", it states in their organization's minutes, "whom the Soc. has declared unworthy of professional fellowship." Although Dr. Geiger had helped write the Society's constitution, when the vote for membership was taken, he was refused admittance to the organization, probably due to his selling patent medicines.

Dr. Crook claimed ignorance to the fact that he was not allowed to consult with anyone outside of the Medical Society and promised not to do so again. This was accepted, but a new resolution was put into place.

Consultation with physicians not members of the Society of doubtful moral and professional standing are derogatory to the best interests of this association by elevating the Quack and justly lowering the true physician in the estimation of the public, and by destroying that distinction which should rather be increased between regular medicine and recent humbug...(it is) resolved that when ever complaint is made by one of this body that a member is in the habit of consulting with any physician not a member of this Society, and of doubtful professional or moral qualifications, this Society shall determine the fact whether such physician is a proper person for members of this association to fellowship with.

Translated, it meant that if a doctor associated with the Society consulted with another doctor who was not, the offending member could be kicked out on his ear. Three months later, at the Society's meeting on January 17, 1858, Dr. Crook was again charged with consulting with Dr. Geiger. This time there was no appeal and Dr. Crook was expelled from the Society.

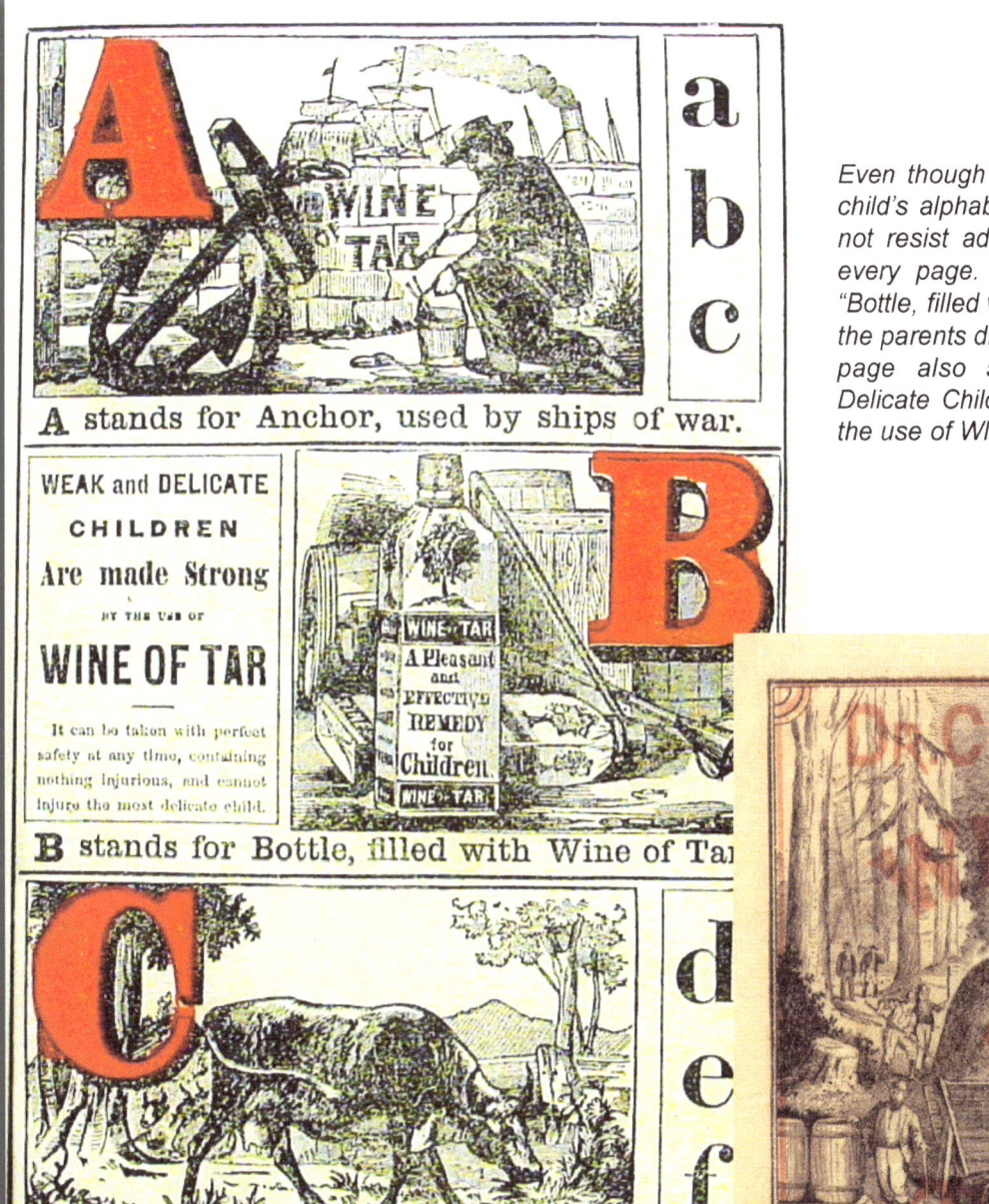

Even though it was supposed to be a child's alphabet book, Dr. Crook could not resist advertising his products on every page. The letter B stood for "Bottle, filled with Wine of Tar." In case the parents didn't get the message, the page also states that "Weak and Delicate Children Are made Strong by the use of WINE OF TAR."

In 1861 Dr. Crook began offering a tonic made of pine tree tar. At first it was called "Dr. Proctor's Wine of Tar" and advertised as being an improvement over the old formula. Who Dr. Proctor was is still a mystery. However, by the end of the Civil War the tonic proved popular enough to be advertised in newspapers outside of Dayton and soon after became known as "Dr. Crook's Wine of Tar". Among its benefits, the ads claimed it could cure consumption, coughs, asthma, diphtheria, sore throat, bronchitis, diabetes, diseases of the kidney - and in case they missed naming your disease - the list ended with the words "and other complaints".

The good doctor also advertised several other remedies, including "Benzoin Elixir" for throat and lung diseases, "Citron Balsam" for curing warts, skin ulcers, gangrene and rheumatism, "S-PH-L-S" for syphilis, "Vegetable Extract" for tumors, old sores and chronic diseases of the eyes, and "Compound Syrup of Poke Root" for everything already mentioned above and claimed to getting rid of pains in the

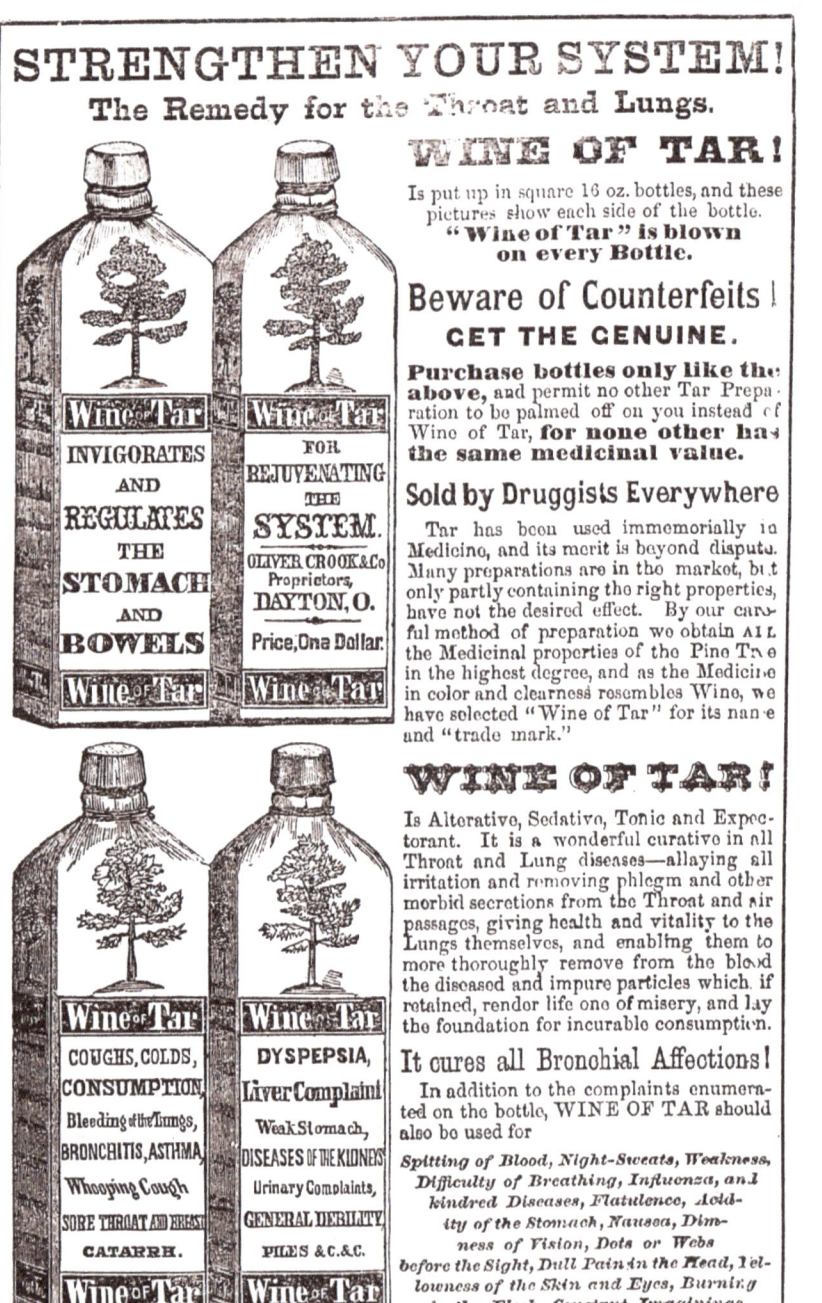
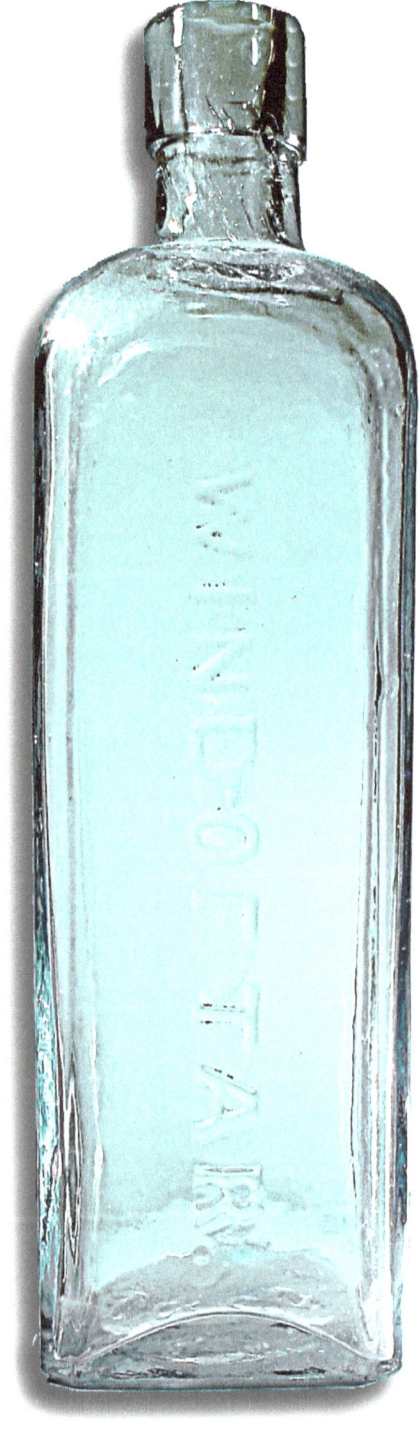

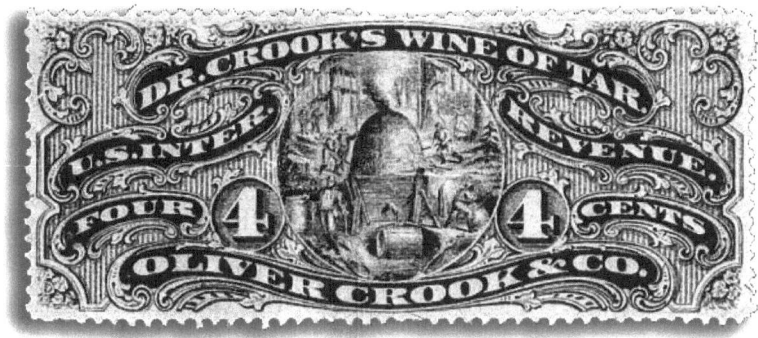

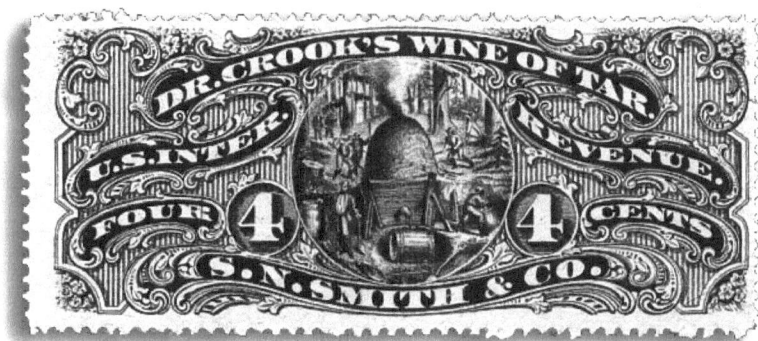

In 1862 a tax law, called the Revenue Act of 1862, was enacted because the Union needed money to fund their part in the Civil War. Among the items taxed were matches, playing cards and patent medicines. The stamps were bought from the government and then placed on the package in such a way that guaranteed that when it was opened the stamp would be torn apart. Manufacturers subject to these taxes were allowed to produce their own stamps. The dies, plates, and reproduction were at the manufacturers' expense, but the dies were controlled by the Treasury. Dr. Oliver Crook eventually availed himself of this free advertising by designing a private die stamp that depicted men in the process of filling a wooden barrel with pine tar, the ingredient in his famous "Wine of Tar" patent medicine. The stamp was issued in March of 1869 and last issued in December of 1875. The Wine of Tar proved to be a popular item, for in that period over 700,000 stamps were issued. When S. N. Smith & Co. took over, the stamp design was altered and reissued in December of 1875 and was last issued on March 27, 1883, the tax having been repealed. Although sales slowed as time passed, another 308,829 stamps were issued, adding up to an estimated purchase of well over one million bottles of Wine of Tar in a fifteen year period.

bones and limbs. By 1871 Dr. Crook had so many remedies that it took an entire column in the newspaper to list them and what they were capable of curing.

Dr. Crook was once described as being dark complexion, sparsely built, and "as lithe and straight as the pine tree from which was distilled the famous Wine of Tar." An indefatigable worker, it was believed that he had the largest practice of any Dayton physician in his day. But the unrelenting work was also his undoing. Dr. Crook died on April 28, 1873 at the age of 54 from complications due to pneumonia.

At the time of his death a request was made in the newspaper for members of the medical profession to meet and make arrangements to attend his death. At the meeting, Dr. Alburtus Geiger gave an impassionate speech about the deceased and the respect the community had for him. Afterwards, the same members of the Medical Society who had turned their backs on Dr. Crook fifteen years before, passed a resolution that they should attend his funeral.

Apparently Dr. Geiger had not exaggerated when he spoke of the town's affection for his deceased friend. Park Presbyterian Church, where the service was held, was quickly filled to capacity. Hundreds of mourners who had been unable to gain entrance remained outside to join the long procession to Woodland Cemetery for his burial there.

Dr. Crook's business partners, Andrew and William E. Gump, William H. Rouzer and Daniel H. Eichelberger, ran the company for about a year after his death. By 1875 it had been bought by S. N. Smith & Co., which consisted of S. N. Smith and John D. Park. Mr. Park, a resident of Cincinnati, dropped out two years later. S. N. Smith continued the business until 1896.

Chapter Five
Dr. Harter Medicine Company

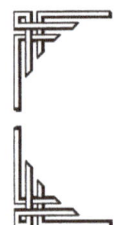
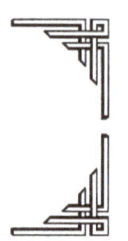

Dr. Milton G. Harter was born in Harrison County, Kentucky in 1817, but at the age of four he moved with his parents to a farm just east of Troy, Ohio. Although he did not attend a public school while growing up, he had a love for learning and resorted to teaching himself. Dr. Harter eventually became an eminent physician, graduating with high honors from several medical institutions, including the Ackley Medical College of Cleveland, Ohio in 1846, the Cincinnati College of Medicine and Surgery of Cincinnati in 1856 and the Bellvue Medical College of New York in 1866. Dr. Harter practiced his profession for several years in Troy, Ohio all the while researching and making new medicines. He first introduced his "Elixir of Wild Cherry" formula in 1855. His first sales did not contain any printing on them, the packages being wrapped in brown paper and personally shipped by the doctor. By 1858 Dr. Harter had moved to Marion, Indiana. It was here that he began manufacturing an ague specific remedy that supposedly cured malaria and miasmatic fevers and sinking

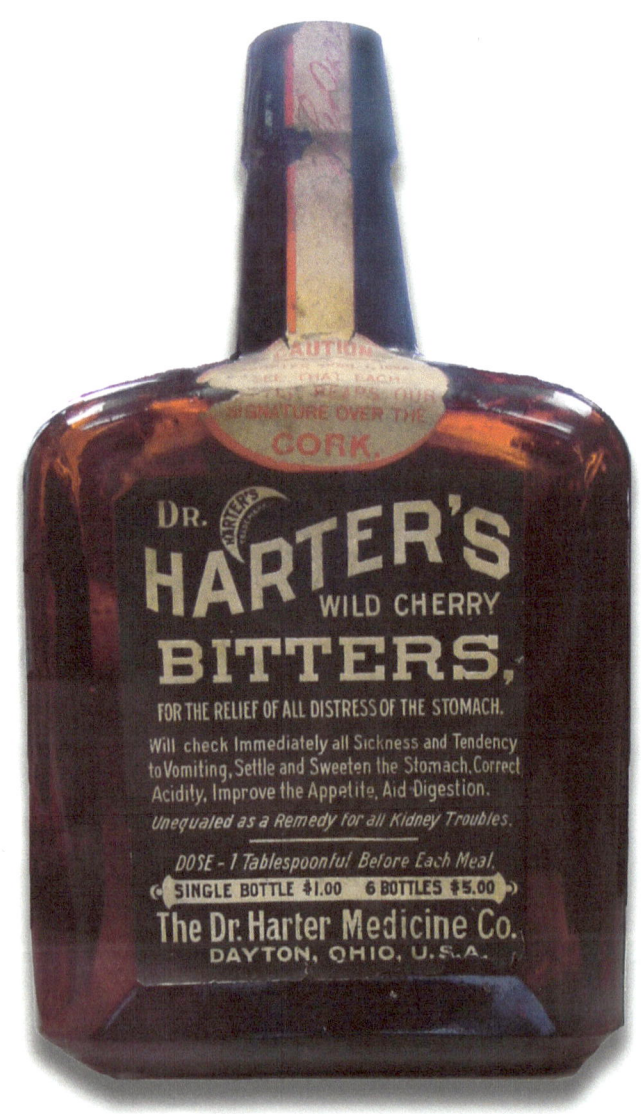

"Harter's Elixir of Wild Cherry", (later renamed Wild Cherry Bitters), had stimulating properties that helped calm the nerves. Its effects were immediate, "causing a gentle glow and warmth throughout the entire body." Its claims included helping sufferers of dyspepsia, all disorders of the stomach and nerves that resulted from overeating and drinking, derangement of the Liver, constipation, languor, headaches "and as a preventative in malarial districts." The company held a design patent on the shape of the bottle.

chills, which did well among the malaria-plagued districts in the Hoosier State. He met with a considerable measure of success at this, but lack of capital stopped him from being able to expand. In 1862 he turned to his brother, Samuel K. Harter, for help. Samuel believed in what his brother was trying to accomplish and agreed to buy a half-interest in the business, which was then moved to Troy. In 1866 the two men established a factory in St. Louis and the Dr. Harter & Company was born. The business ran under that name for several years. After Milton died in 1872 Samuel incorporated the business, which then became known as the Dr. Harter Medicine Company.

In 1895 Samuel found himself turning 72 years old. He longed to come back to his boyhood stomping grounds in Troy. In order to move the business to Ohio from Missouri, it became necessary to for Samuel to form a co-partnership, including as managing members William M. Hayner (Samuel Harter's son-in-law) and Walter S. Kidder (William M. Hayner's brother-in-law).

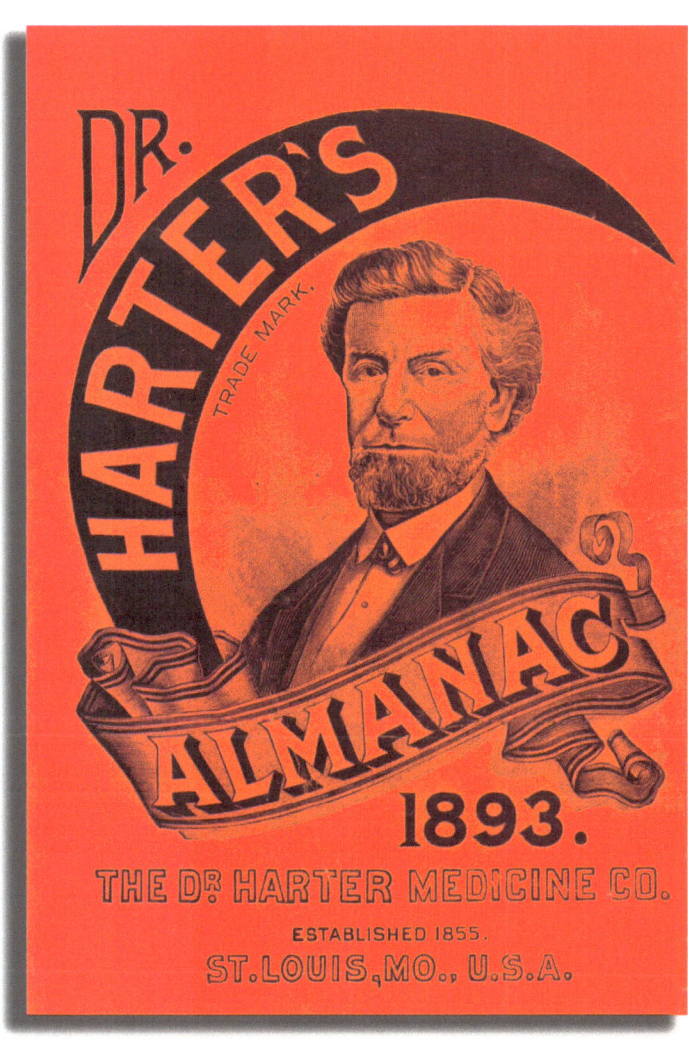

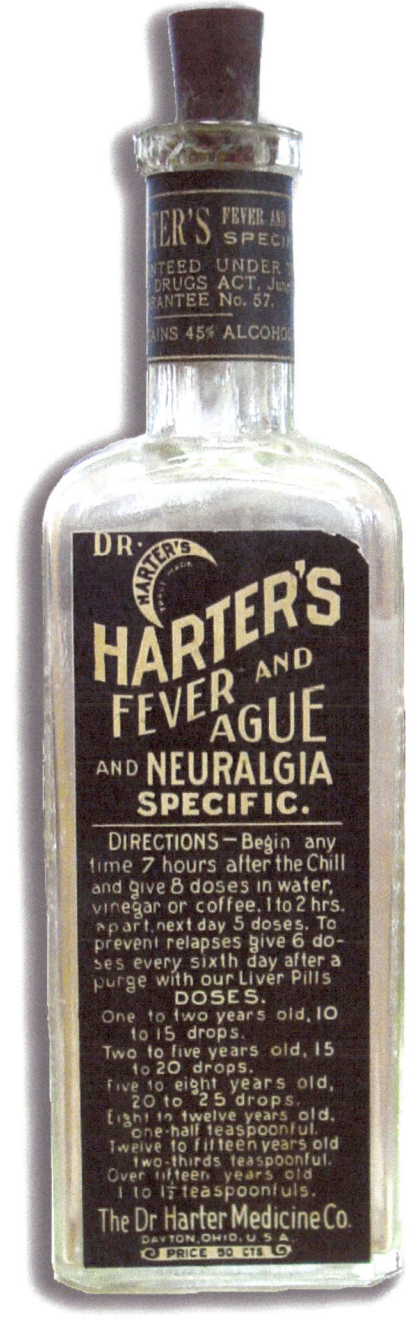

Above: Dr. Milton G. Harter graced the cover of the company's advertisements and literature for years after his death in 1872.

Right: Harter's Fever, Ague and Neuralgia Specific. A "No Cure, No Pay!" guarantee accompanied each bottle. The remedy gave relief to sufferers of fever and ague, intermittent fever, neuralgia, marsh and swamp fevers, malaria and miasmatic fevers, sinking chills, and more if taken according to directions.

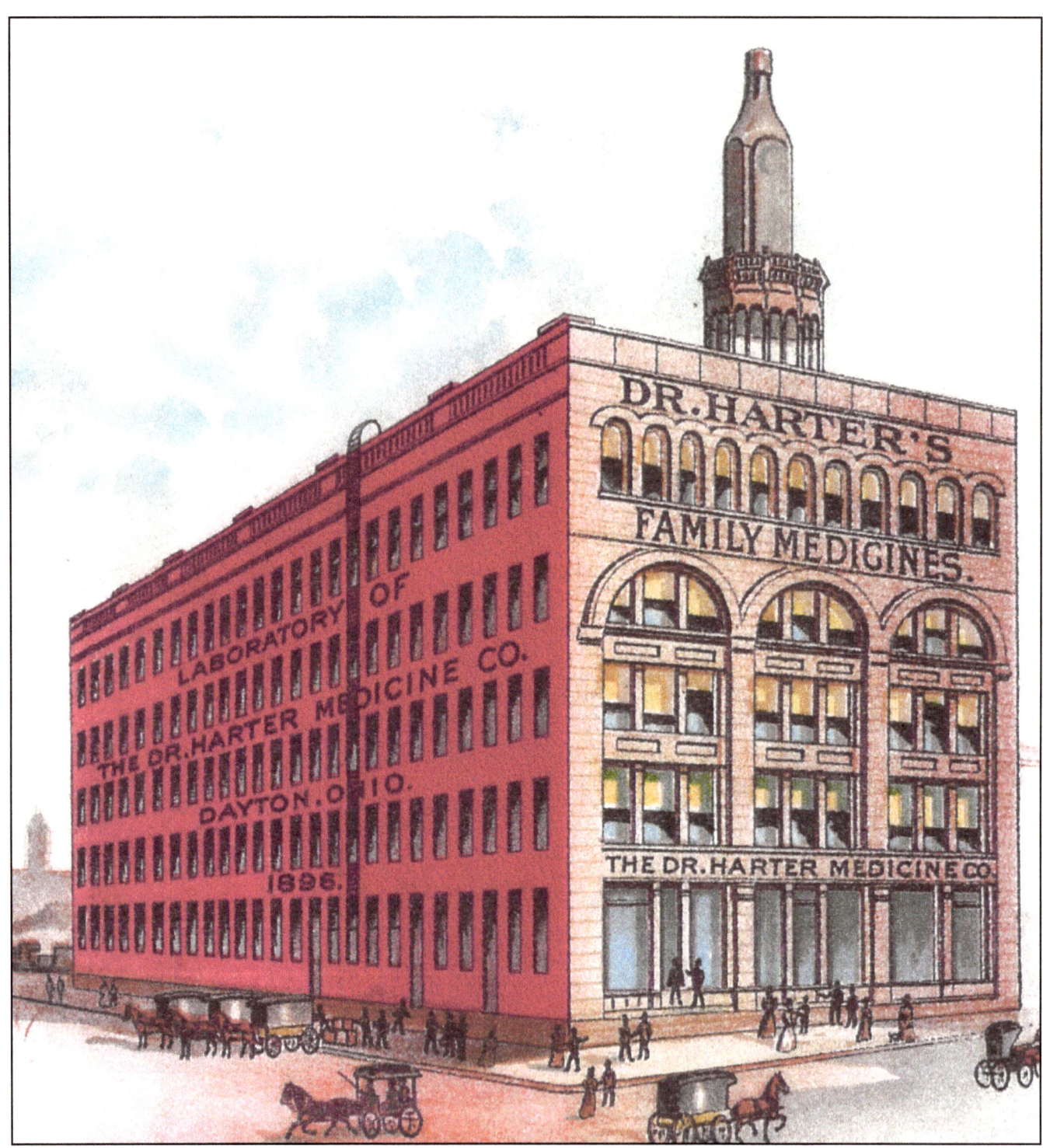

The 180 x 50 foot structure extended along the Miami & Erie canal. The first floor was used for office and shipping, the second for packing, the fourth for bottling and the third and fifth for labeling. A vast printing department filled the basement. The wooden bottle sitting on top of the building was not only advertisement, but also acted as a water tower.

Several cities around Troy begged for the Dr. Harter Medicine Company to relocate in their area, but Dayton was the most logical choice. The city was close to Troy and was big enough to be able to handle the 20 million pieces of printing material the company distributed each year, as well as the transportation of their product across the United States. A site was secured at what is now the northeast corner of Monument and Patterson Boulevard, the canal then running along where the Boulevard is now. A five story, pressed brick building with over 70,000 feet of floor space was erected, making it one of the largest medicine manufacturing plants in the country. In case anyone wondered what was going on inside, a huge wooden medicine bottle was placed on top of the building which could be seen for blocks around.

The day of August 5, 1895 was set aside as a holiday in Dayton, to celebrate the coming of the first train carrying equipment and staff for the new business. A large delegation of Dayton businessmen also traveled to St. Louis to accompany the train back to the Gem City. When the train arrived at the Union Depot at 4:10 p.m., all of the whistles of the factories in Dayton began to blow and the Central fire station bell was rung, signaling thousands of people to gather to help the Dayton Board of Trade greet the Harter party.

Soon the streets were crowded to capacity in order to watch a parade. Starting with a platoon of mounted police, the demonstration included hundreds of express wagons and carriages, as well as wagons from the Harter Company. All of the vehicles were covered with Roman candles and red lights; one observer stating that parade looked like "a line of fire."

A banquet followed at the Hotel Atlas, where almost 150 of Dayton's best citizens gathered to toast the city's newest enterprise. A representative for the Harter Medicine Company was quoted as saying during the dinner that, while he had been informed that the population did not exceed 80,000 citizens, he felt sure he had counted 800,000 people when the train reached Dayton.

Even while the festivities were going on downtown, workmen were busy emptying the eighteen railroad cars of equipment into the new Harter building. The following morning the doors were thrown open and the work of manufacturing was underway. A few days later gaudily painted wagons bearing the Harter name, and the city of its manufacturing as Dayton, started out on their deliveries throughout the country.

The company produced a wide variety of products, including "Harter's Elixir of Wild Cherry", (later renamed "Wild Cherry Bitters"), "Fever, Ague and Neuralgia Specific", "Harter's Liniment", "Harter's Iron Tonic" and "Harter's Lung Balm" to name just a few. There was even (no fooling) "Harter's Little Liver Pills".

The Dr. Harter Medicine Company registered a number of trademarks, including the crescent that carried the name Harter's name in the new moon and the word Dr. above. The company also held a design patent on their Wild Cherry's rectangular amber bottle.

The Harter Company didn't seem to be shy when it came to protecting its copyrights, even stating in their literature that anyone sending in information leading to the conviction of companies infringing on their patents would be "liberally rewarded." By 1893 the company had sued and obtained judgment against thirty-two individuals for various copyright infringements, including two in 1889 confirming both the patent on the Wild Cherry's bottle and the crescent trademark found on all of the companies labels and products.

When Samuel Harter died in June 1898 William Hayner and Walter Kidder decided to sell the business and turn their full attention to the Hayner Distilling Company, a whiskey distillery in Troy owned by William's family. On November 1, 1900 The Doctor Harter Medicine Co. was incorporated yet again, this time with B. H. Winters as President and Oscar F. Davisson as Vice-President. The Dr. Harter Medicine Company held on in Dayton for another decade, but by 1911 it was no longer in Dayton, being bought out by the C. I. Hood Company, out of Massachusetts.

Dayton was not to lose her crown as a well-known provider of proprietary medicines, however. It wasn't long before a new sign was afloat atop the old Harter building, as we will see in the next chapter.

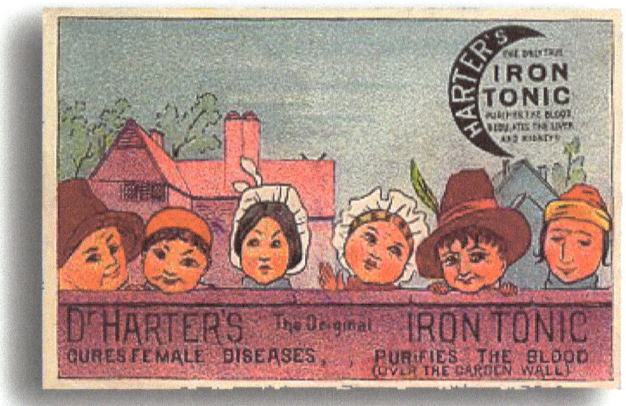

Harter's Iron Tonic, originally called "Magic Tonic", would eventually become one of the top sellers in patent medicine. The tonic claimed many things, including giving the taker strength, improving the appetite and purifying the blood, curing dropsy, neuralgia and even epilepsy. The tonic contained pyrophosphate iron, which was thought to help digest food and build up blood cells.

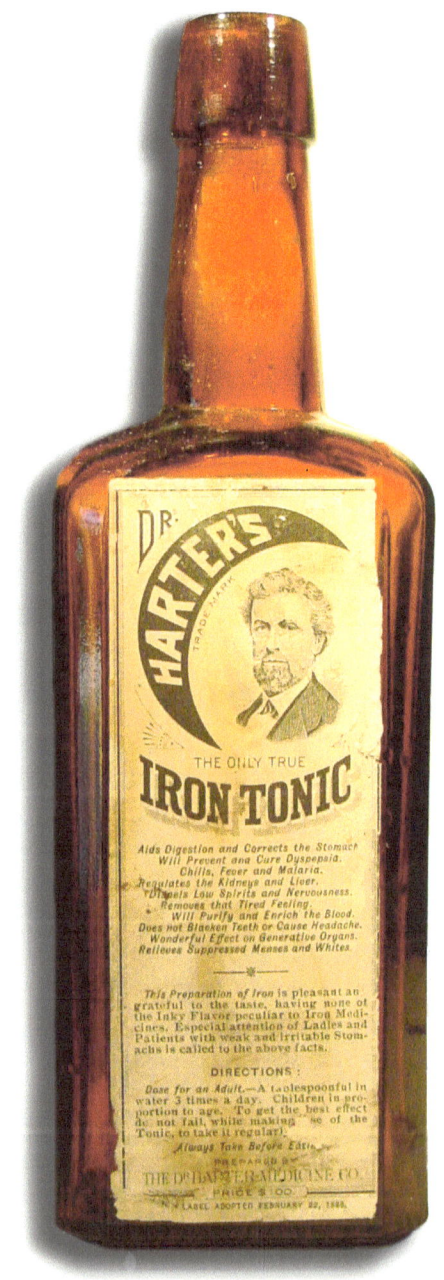
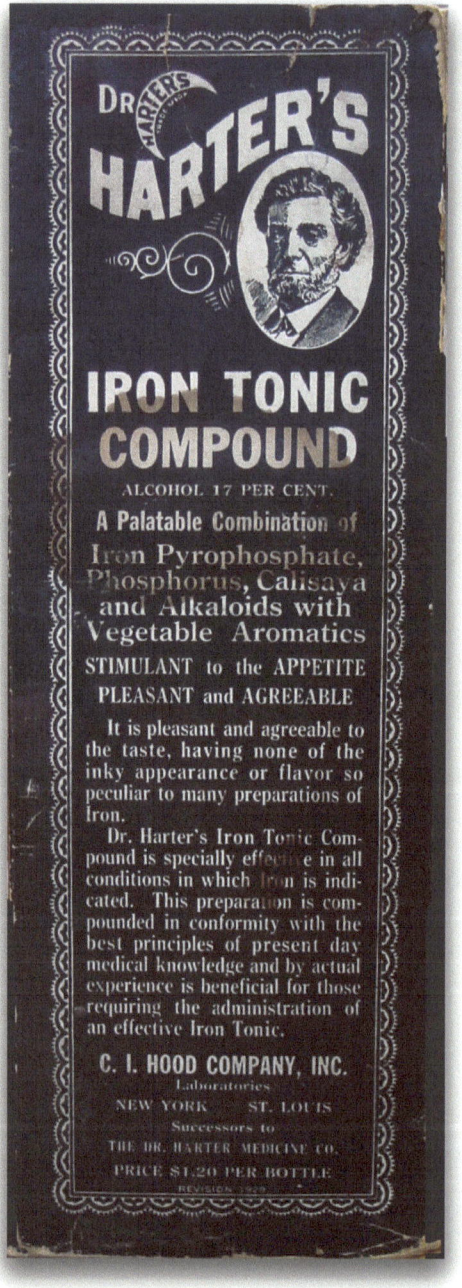

Chapter Six
Cooper Medicine Company

Even as the Dr. Harter Medicine Company began to decline at the turn of the century another nostrum manufacturer was on the rise in the Gem City.

Lee T. Cooper was born in Germantown, Kentucky May 11, 1875, his parents being James and Mary Cooper. While hardly more than a boy he became a salesman for the Sun Life Insurance company in Lexington. At the age of 17 he won a gold medal for selling more insurance than any other agent in the company, a talent that would later prove useful.

The way Lee told it, the Cooper Medicine Company actually began with the death of his uncle, Dr. G. H. Cooper, a famous physician and chemist in New York City. When he died, Dr. Cooper decided to leave Lee the formula of a preparation which he had spent years perfecting, and with which he had obtained remarkable results in the treatment of stomach, kidney and liver diseases.

Lee immediately decided to continue on with his uncle's work. He contacted his brothers, Jesse and William R. Cooper, and in the winter of 1900-01 they built a small laboratory in a room at 812 East Fifth Street in Dayton, Ohio. The company was soon churning out bottles of "Cooper's New Discovery".

In order to get the word out about their new product, the brothers decided to take to the road and travel to towns unfamiliar with their remedies. Lee decided to use a mammoth band wagon, drawn by six prancing horses, to lead his caravan. Everyone along the roads couldn't help but notice the immense plate mirrors blazing with hundreds of tiny incandescent lamps, or the top which could seat a forty-piece band.

When the caravan reached its destination, a large space of ground would be rented and a platform erected to act as a stage for the performers. In the background a stage curtain separated the stage from the dressing room. The whole place would take on the feel of a carnival as tents were erected nearby to feed and house the company's staff.

The real activity began at sundown. The brass band would strike up popular tunes of the day and soon the townspeople would gather to find out what all the fuss was about. They would soon discover a stage brightly illuminated by a number of gasoline chandeliers and the players of a vaudeville or musical act taking the stage, who would entertain the crowd for free.

The action between the performances was no less entertaining. Lee would quickly take the platform in a long English walking coat, diamonds on his lapels, five and ten dollar gold coins for buttons. In a voice like that of an old-time revivalist, Lee would loudly explain the nature of the different diseases and the virtues of the Cooper remedies. One such story told of how, while traveling in "Old

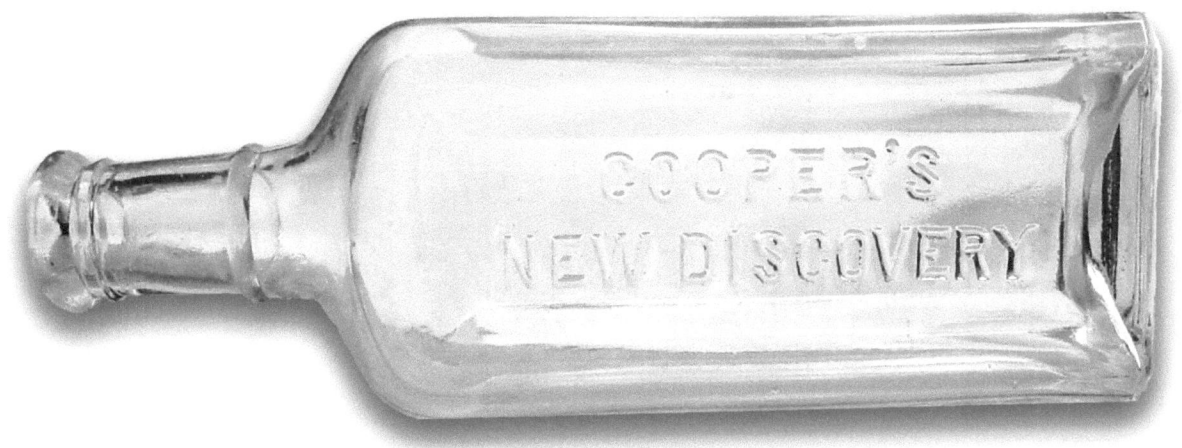

Mexico", Lee purchased from an old Spanish priest the formula for a liniment which was claimed by the natives there to possess almost miraculous powers. Finding this to be true, Lee began manufacturing the ointment under the name "Cooper's Quick Relief". He would then invite from the audience "all sufferers of pain" to receive a free treatment to prove that "quick relief" from whatever ailed them was just a dollar away.

To the astonishment of those gathered, people who were deaf for years were suddenly made to hear, stiff joints and limbs were quickly limbered up, toothache and rheumatic pains were instantly dispelled by the application of this preparation.

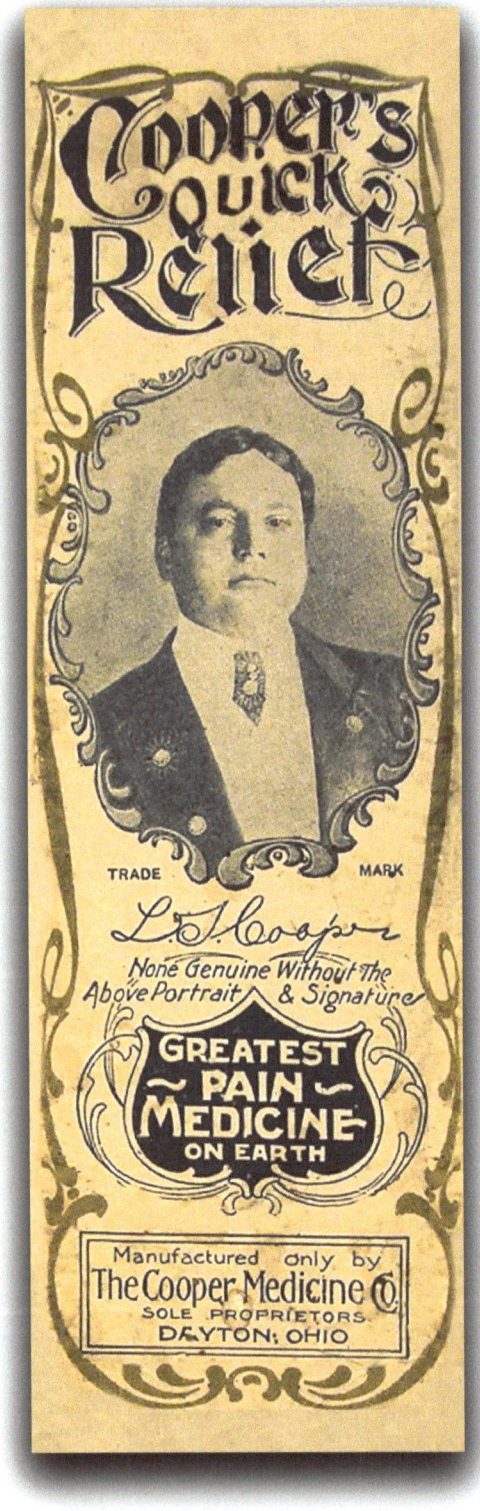

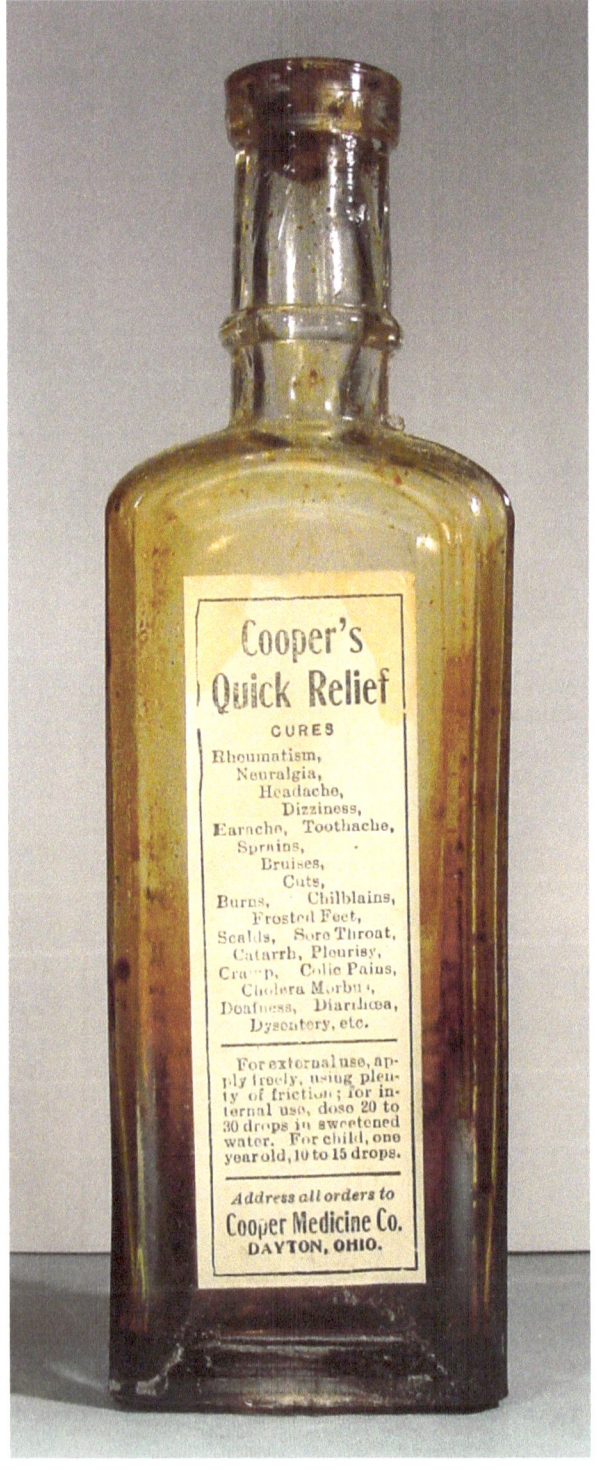

After these "miracles", bottles of "Cooper's New Discovery" were quickly brought out, and the good Dr. Cooper would explain about the years his uncle spent creating a medicine that works on the insides, treating "that dreaded disease so few in our country are free from, catarrh" (inflammation of the mucous membranes).

Lee advanced the theory that catarrh affected different vital parts of the body and such diseases as stomach, liver and kidney diseases, rheumatism and "impure blood" are afflictions that he claimed could be cured by buying a bottle of "New Discovery." In fact, Lee was so sure that it would cure whatever ailed the buyer that each package came with a guarantee to give perfect satisfaction or all money would be refunded.

Besides the brass band, Lee had other ways of spreading the word that he was in town. One day a reporter standing on a street in Lexington, Kentucky noticed hundreds of people passing by, each with loaves of bread in their hands.

There were so many bearing the 'staff of life' that my curiosity was aroused. I stepped to a man I presumed to be a native and asked: "Did everybody in Lexington run out of bread at the same time?" "No, not that," was the smiling reply. "There's a medicine man on a vacant lot down the street by the name of Cooper and before he starts his show each night he gives away hundreds of loaves of bread to the poorer classes of the city."

Sometimes the gimmick involved a parade. The local newspapers would be told ahead of time that the Cooper Medicine show would be coming to town and that the caravan would be traveling down the main thoroughfare. Dr. Lee T. Cooper (all of the brothers seemed to use the term 'doctor' liberally while on the road) would confide to the reporter that his parade was going to cause a sensation. When asked why, Dr. Cooper would reply that he would be throwing small items to the people lined up along the street, as was customary in those days. Why a sensation? Lee answered that question for readers of the Coshocton Daily Age newspaper just before his show opened there on June 30, 1903.

I shall have $200 in a grip in my carriage and it will be filled with not only dimes and nickels, but quarters, halves and dollars as well. I shall throw these coins by the handful into the crowds. I hardly believe there will be any left for the street sweeping gang next morning.

Although the shows were held in the evening, the daylight hours were not wasted. Cooper would rent an office, or set up a tent if necessary, and consult with patients. Within a day or two of seeing the miracles he was performing on stage, townspeople would soon line up for private consultations. You could rest assured that the treatment for their ailments usually involved a case or two of Cooper's New Discovery.

After three weeks or so, sales would begin to dry up and it would be time to go back to Dayton, fill up the wagon, and move on to the next rubes, uh, town. A final farewell would be arranged to try and clear up what bottles still remained. The last night would usually promise to have a wood sawing contest between two women, the winner taking home $3. That was different enough to get the crowds to gather one last time. After the contest was over, baskets full of groceries would be brought on stage and the crowd told to quiet down. An announcement would be made, stating that, astonishingly, a basket of groceries would be given away with each $3 purchase of medicine. Six bottles and two baskets could be had for five dollars; a ten-spot would be good for twelve bottles and four baskets full of groceries. Excitement was enhanced by claiming the sale was strictly on a first-come, first served basis and only while supplies lasted.

In an article titled "Mad Rush to Get Medicine" an observer wrote of what usually happened next.

Some of the baskets, at least, contained only a peck of potatoes and a loaf of bread. There was a wild stampede, however, to get up to the platform and hand over the cash. The doctor took all that came, perhaps as a memento of his visit. He had the people perfectly wild, and sold his medicine in $10 lots. It is estimated that Dr. Cooper left about $5,000 richer than when he came here about three weeks ago.

But articles berating the Cooper Medicine show were rare. Instead, stories circulated of how Dr.

Cooper took a deaf man up onto the platform and within three minutes of placing drops in his ears, the man could hear the doctor snap his fingers from twenty feet away. It seemed miraculous, but the stories appeared again and again.

So, did Cooper Medicine really have a cure for deafness? Well, sort of. Many people of that day and age with hearing problems had nothing more serious than impacted ear wax. A few drops of oil or glycerin to soften it up, the use of a cloth or a tilt of the head to remove the oil and wax, and suddenly the deaf could hear again. It also helped that many of Cooper's ads were made to look like newspaper articles. With headings in bold type shouting "DEAF TWENTY YEARS BUT NOW THEY HEAR - Miraculous Cures Wrought by Dr. Cooper and His Magical Medicines", who couldn't help but read them, or believe them?

The medicine show business didn't always go smoothly. One summer Jesse Cooper, who had been selling medicine in West Uhrichsville for several weeks, was arrested by the local Marshall, on a warrant sworn out by Frank Winders, secretary of the state board of medical examiners. Winders charged that Jesse was practicing medicine without a license. Later the prisoner was released after he assured the Marshall that he administered the medicine under the direction of Dr. E. C. Bell, a regularly licensed physician who was accompanying the show.

In February 1902, Cooper Medicine Company incorporated with Lee Cooper as acting President. Lee's brother, Joseph, joined in the venture soon after as secretary. Business was booming and a decision was made to move the laboratories to 113 East Second Street, which offered eight times more floor space. Beginning in 1903 Lee still visited the larger cities to give personal demonstrations, but had turned to lecturing in auditoriums, his audience numbering close to eight thousand a night.

Lee Cooper was well-known for his generosity, especially when it came to less-fortunate children. Unfortunately, one act of kindness that ended in tragedy would continue to haunt him for years.

While giving a lecture in Indianapolis, Lee Cooper invited 600 newspaper boys to attend a free performance on April 17th, 1905 at the Unique Theater on East Washington Street. He reminded them that they had to have a ticket to attend, which could be picked up at the local Masonic Temple.

Long before the time appointed for the distribution of the tickets, the stairs to the Masonic Temple were crowded with a pushing, yelling crowd of young boys, each anxious to make sure that he got a pass. When the actual distribution began, the excitement became even more intense. Policemen who had been detailed to prevent trouble soon lost control.

A witness to the scene later claimed that one of the boys, probably in an effort to get closer to the front of the line, shouted "Fire!" Immediately those at the top turned around and began to force their way to the bottom of the stairs. Shrieks and fighting soon began among the frightened boys, with some of those near the top falling headlong upon the struggling mass at the bottom.

Police responded to a call that a riot was occurring at the Temple. The boys were disentangled as fast as possible, but the policemen and ambulance crews were hampered in their work by an immense crowd of people from the business district who jostled around at the bottom the stairs. Even with the aid of at least fifty police, doctors and rescuers, it required over three-quarters of an hour to remove everyone from the stairwell. Blood trickled down the steps and fragments of clothing were strewn everywhere.

Due to the sheer number of injured, the boys had to be taken to different hospitals and dispensaries, and men had to be stationed at these institutions to keep family members from breaking into the rooms where the youngsters were being treated.

In the end, four boys had died: Ed Morrissey, 12 years old; Floyd Poland, 8; Louis Scheigert, 15; and Homer Williamson, 11. Over one hundred others were injured in the crush.

A week later, damage suits were filed in Federal Court at Cincinnati by the parents of the four boys. The defendants in each case were the Cooper Medicine Company and Lee T. Cooper, asking for $5,000 in damages. The complaints charged that the defendants were guilty of gross neglect in failing to provide for the care and management of the estimated 1,000 boys who were thought to have gathered to get a ticket.

The case dragged through the Indiana, Ohio and Federal courts for several years. It wasn't until December 18, 1911 that Judge Howard Hollister, of the United States District Court, had the final word and dismissed the suits.

By autumn of 1905 the company found it necessary to move into even larger quarters. Fortunately for them, room was available in the Dr. Harter's Medicine Company building at the corner of First and Canal streets. The business eventually took over most of the five floors after Dr. Harter's moved out two years later. Joseph Cooper, along with John T. Foote and Joseph Trimbach, also began running a company called Approved Formula from the same location. Less than ten years later the company moved to even larger headquarters at 301-309 East Fifth Street.

In 1915 the Cooper Medicine Company began a marketing campaign for a new medicine, and soon the whole country was talking about Tanlac and hopping to the nearest drug store to get it. Tanlac was advertised to be made of roots, barks and herbs from the most remote corners of the world. These special ingredients would be shipped to Dayton and mixed under the watchful eye of a renowned chemist from Germany. The exotic blend would be bottled and another batch of Tanlac would be on its way to consumers across the land.

The first bottle of Tanlac was sold in Lexington, Kentucky around the beginning of 1915. By March 1918 G. F. Willis, a distributor in Atlanta, Georgia, sent in an order for 335,200 bottles to be shipped for distribution. By November of that same year, it was reported that the company has sold over 1 million bottles through various distributors across the US.

The popularity of Tanlac eventually became noticed by both the press and the medical community. At the turn of the century, journalists began exposing nostrums laden with harmful ingredients, as well as those they considered having no use whatsoever. The most influential work was a ten article series by Samuel Hopkins Adams that first appeared in Collier's on October 7, 1905, entitled *The Great American Fraud*. The American Medical Association picked up the cause and began a campaign against the patent medicine business. Numerous articles began appearing in the *Journal of the American Medical Association* dealing with patent medicine fraud. These articles were reprinted over the years in book form. Titled *Nostrums and Quackery*, the volumes were issued by the Association in 1911, 1921, and 1936. Unfortunately for Lee, the Cooper Medicine Company was criticized quite heavily in the second volume. It spoke of how both "Cooper's New Discovery" and "Cooper's Quick Relief" had been declared misbranded under the Pure Food and Drugs Act. Chemists working for the Federal government reported that the "New Discovery" contained 20 per cent alcohol, some emodin (a laxative derived from plants), aloes and a small quantity of oil of sassafras with reducing sugars. The claim that the tonic was an effective treatment for the diseases of kidneys, blood diseases, diabetes and the like was declared recklessly and wantonly false and fraudulent under the act. The "Quick Relief" also came under fire. The liniment was found to consist of cayenne pepper in 31 per cent alcohol that was flavored with sassafras. The claim that it would afford instant relief to sprains and pain and was a remedy for croup and effective for preventing injuries due to burns and scalds from becoming inflamed was also declared false and fraudulent. A notice of Judgment was issued on November 13, 1916 and the company was fined $50 and costs.

The American Medical Association's book also included twelve pages devoted to the company's tonic, "Tanlac." The article immediately lets the reader know that there was no love lost between the Association and Lee Cooper.

Tanlac is a product of the Cooper Medicine Company, Dayton, Ohio. The controlling spirit of the Cooper concern seems to be one L. T. Cooper, who has been quacking it for many years. A few years ago it was "Cooper's New Discovery" that was being exploited by L. T. Cooper by the free vaudeville-medicine-show route. In 1907 Cooper was operating the "tapeworm trick" as one of his means of relieving the gullible of their money... "Catarrh" is Cooper's catchword. Every ailment is "catarrh" and the one infallible cure for "catarrh" is - according to Cooper - Tanlac!

The Association had bought a bottle of the product and conducted tests on its contents in its Chemical Laboratory. They concluded that Tanlac was essentially a wine flavored with wild cherry, to which had been added some bitter herbs, a small amount of laxative and some glycerin. An alcohol content of 16 per cent was what gave the tonic its "kick."

To add insult to injury, much of the article concentrated on how some of the testimonials stating how great Tanlac was had been falsified, or had been given by people who died soon thereafter.

Lee Cooper had had enough and decided to sell the business. By January 1921 it was owned by the newly formed International Proprietaries, Inc. The company continued to use the Dayton location as a manufacturing plant until sometime around the beginning of World War II.

Lee turned his attention to real estate developments in and around Dayton, Ohio and Miami, Florida. Horse racing was his favorite sport and he owned a string of fast-steppers that made history on many tracks. "El Portal," an attractive suburb of Miami, was promoted by Lee. He took a loss when he later attempted to open a gigantic horse race track in southern Florida he had named "Pompano." But he tired of this as well, and eventually began disposing of the land he owned.

It was front-page news when, less than six years later, Lee Thomas Cooper died on December 17, 1927 following an emergency operation for gallbladder trouble. His obituary made note of how Lee was well known for his generosity, including helping less fortunate boys obtain college degrees. Lee was laid to rest in Woodland Cemetery.

Although nostrums would continue to be made for years to come, the age of the self-made, flamboyant medicine men had come to an end.

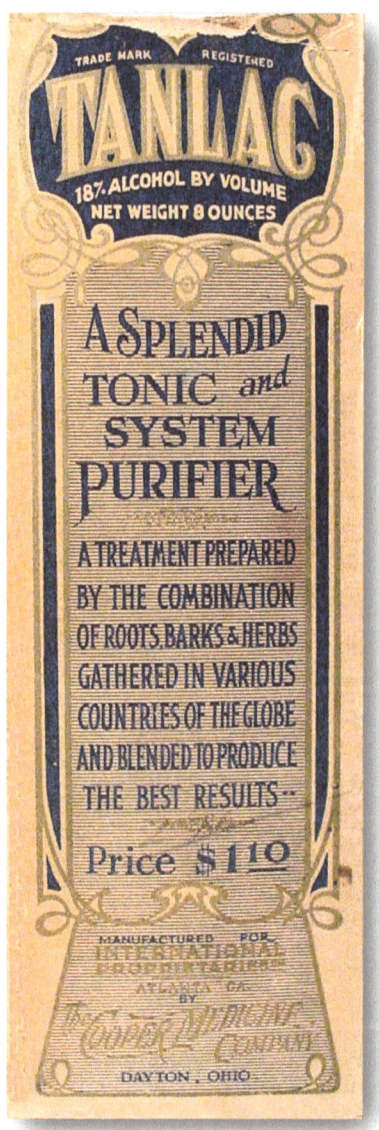
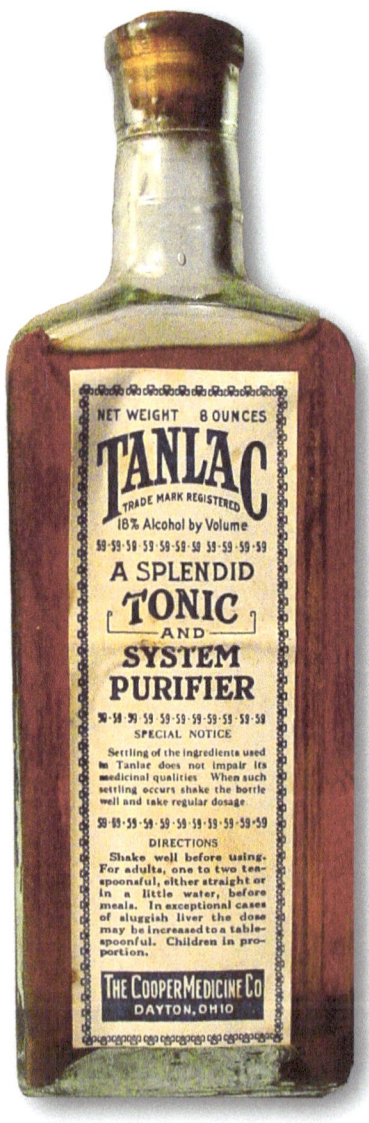

After a time, International Proprietaries, Inc. no longer advertised Tanlac as a "system purifier" but simply as a "stomachic tonic." The alcohol content was dropped to 10% and iron, thiamin and niacin were added. The label gave directions for use by children 6 to 12 years old, the dose being a teaspoon diluted in a half-glass of water. It was not to be given to children under the age of six.

Attack of the Parasites

Nothing would seem scarier for the average person than to think that his or her woes might be due to an eighty foot long tapeworm inside their intestines. Unfortunately, in the days of undercooked meat, tapeworms were a real problem. Several Dayton nostrum sellers took advantage of this fear.

The Dr. Harter Medicine Company's remedy was called "German Vermifuge Candy." According to Dr. Harter, if not taken care of, worms would "produce spasms, impair the health, injure the system, destroy the mind and cause insanity." And since children are reluctant to take medicine, the company prepared the medicine in the form of a great tasting candy "so that the smallest child would gladly take it, and cry for more." Parents were told to look for the warning signs that their children might be suffering from worms; the symptoms included bad breath, restlessness in sleeping and picking their nose.

DR. HARTER'S VERMIFUGE CANDY.
WORMS,
The most common disease, and one to which every child is subject, can be removed by the use of **Dr. Harter's Vermifuge Candy.**
CAUSE MUCH SUFFERING,
Produce spasms, impair the health, injure the system, destroy the mind and cause insanity. The dislike children have to taking medicine, induced Dr. Harter to prepare it in the form of **Candy,** so that the smallest child would gladly take it, and cry for more. This remedy is safe, certain and pleasant, and is sure to give satisfaction.
CHILDREN
troubled with worms will usually show it by one or more symptoms, such as Sleep Restless, Grinds the Teeth, Picks the Nose, Fever, Lips and Abdomen Swollen, Bad Breath, etc., which can be cured by **Dr. Harter's Vermifuge Candy.** Directions on each bottle. Price, 25 cents.

Among the other preparations that could be found were the "Dr. H. F. Weis Tape Worm Remedy" and "Dr. Weis' Worm Salve", "Ka-Vita" was offered up by the Dayton Medicine Company, and several manufacturers of "cure-alls" included the treatment of worms in among their various other promises.

But no one from Dayton used the dread of worms to their advantage as well as Lee. T. Cooper did. Testimonials and newspaper stories spread the word of how just a few doses of "Cooper's New Discovery" were ridding people of 75, 100 and even 125 feet long tape worms that had been sapping their life away. One case in 1905 involved a Toledo woman by the name of Miss L. Wentworth who, after taking seven doses of Cooper's medicine, passed a parasite eighty feet long. She had supposedly taken the still alive and squirming worm to Lee Cooper in a glass jar in order to find out what it was. After telling her that her troubles were over, he persuaded the woman to let him exhibit the parasite outside his office, where thousands of the city's residents popped by to take a gander at it.

The truth is, although Cooper's medicine very well could have been the reason the parasites being expelled, many of the specimens displayed by patent medicine showmen across the country had probably never seen the inside of a human. The abnormally large tapeworms were usually purchased by the nostrum dealers from the local slaughterhouse, the worms being taken from the insides of cattle.

When the Cooper Medicine Show arrived in Cochocton, Ohio in the summer of 1903, an enterprising grocery store in the city created this unusual ad, claiming that it, too, had everything a person needed to cure what ailed them, including stomach troubles, rheumatism and tapeworms.

McCABE'S MARKET
Feed your tape worms on our ice cream. It will give as much relief as Cooper's remedy.
Our fruit tablets cure all stomach troubles.
Our Lemons are a sure cure for rheumatism.
Our watermelons cure all malarial diseases.
One quart of our Peanuts eaten before retiring insures a good night's rest.
A prominent man, who does not want his name mentioned, has just removed a 90 ft. tape worm by feeding it 10 lbs of our salted pop corn.
Bell 'Phone 483   **E. A. M'CABE**   553 Main Street
A. M. D. O. F. F. F.

Chapter Seven
Druggists

The pharmacies of the nineteenth century in Dayton weren't what we think of them as today. In addition to compounding medicines from doctor's prescriptions, many times the drug stores handled paints, varnishes, glassware, and even hard liquor, the latter carried for "medicinal" purposes. Nostrum manufacturers like Lee T. Cooper helped popularize patent medicines to the point that people asked for them by name and it behooved pharmacies to carry their products. Some of the pharmacists in Dayton, seeing how well these medicines were selling, decided to hop on the patent medicine wagon, too. After all, since they filled prescriptions for physicians, most of the drug stores were already carrying the ingredients they needed to make their own concoctions.

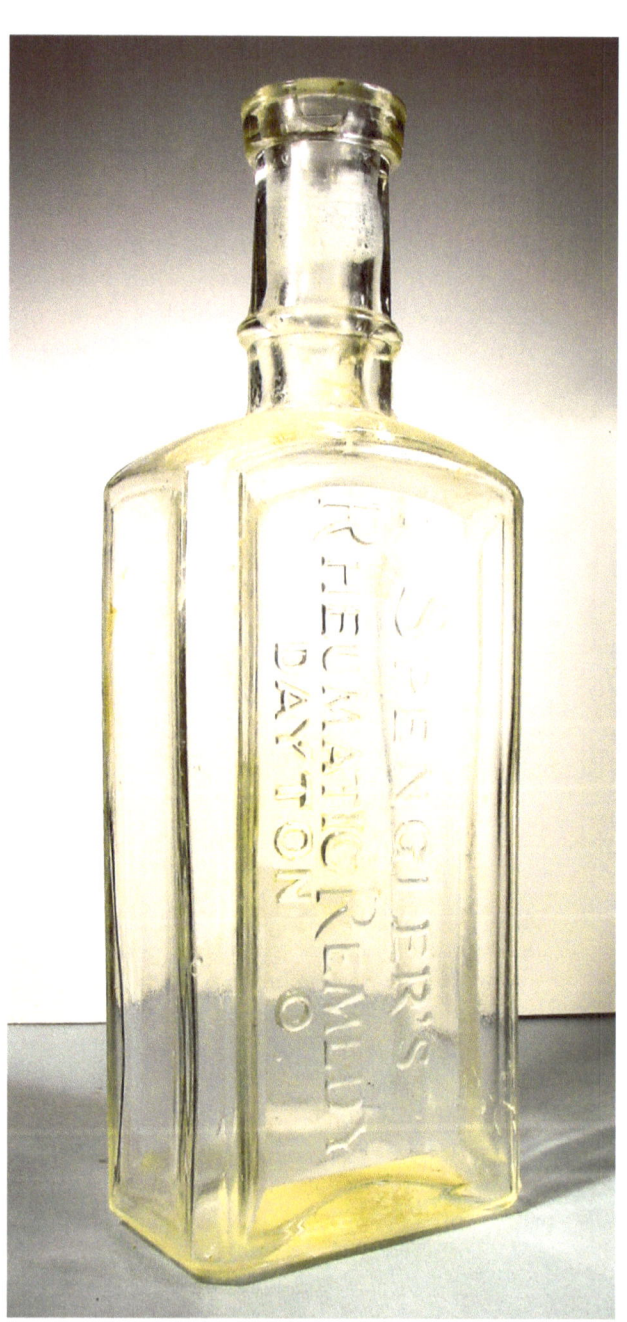

Spengler's Drug Store

John G. Spengler owned a drug store on the northeast corner of Second and Webster Street. In 1897 he began offering his customers a cure for rheumatism. Called Spengler's Rheumatic Remedy, the elixir sold for seventy-five cents a bottle, not bad considering other remedies of the time usually sold for at least a dollar. Although not a national best-seller by any means, Spengler's mixture did prove popular enough for other drug stores in the area to carry on their shelves. Although Spengler's pharmacy continued to thrive for many years, for reasons now lost in time, Spengler seems to have discontinued his remedy soon after the end of World War I.

RHEUMATISM can be easily helped and the pain relieved by using a remedy that has done so for hundreds of our people. It is sold by all Druggists. Made in Dayton and endorsed by all who have used it. Just USE **SPENGLER'S RHEUMATIC REMEDY**

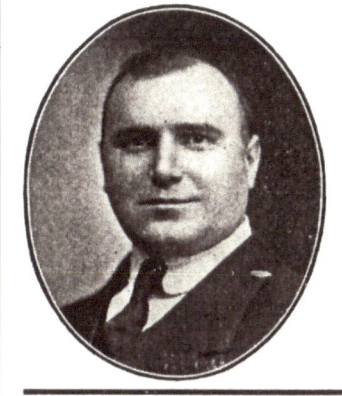

Wietzel Drug Company

Christopher J. Wietzel started a pharmacy at the corner of Fifth and Brown Streets in 1900. By 1909 Wietzel's motto was "Everything in Drugs", which included several that he made himself. One of his most popular was named "Wietzel's Stomach and Bowel Tonic." The preparation was very efficient when used to regulate the bowels, but also had the side effect of improving the appetitie, promoting digestion, relieving heartburn, settling an upset stomach and even clearing up the users complextion. The tonic came in two sizes, a small bottle could be bought for fifty cents, a larger bottle cost one dollar.

Wietzel's other products included a remedy that helped sufferers of bronchitis and an expectorant cold tablet that helped clear the lungs and stop coughs.

For a short time in the mid 1940's Wietzel also offered "Zelax Indian Herb Tablets." Made of all natural ingredients, including dandelion and rhubarb, the tablets supposedly helped stimulate the liver and relieve constipation and sick headaches.

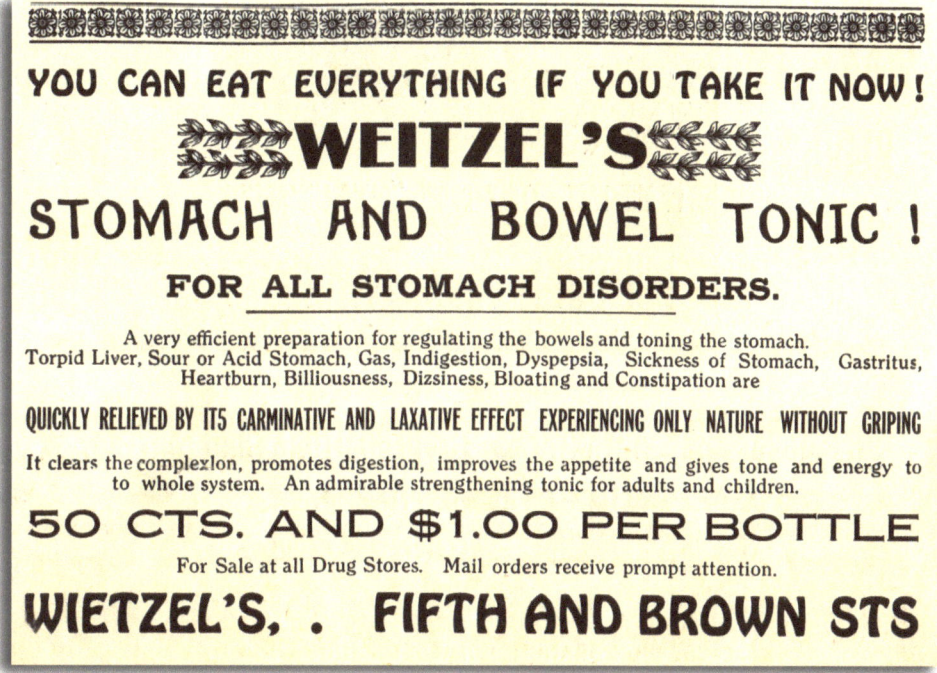

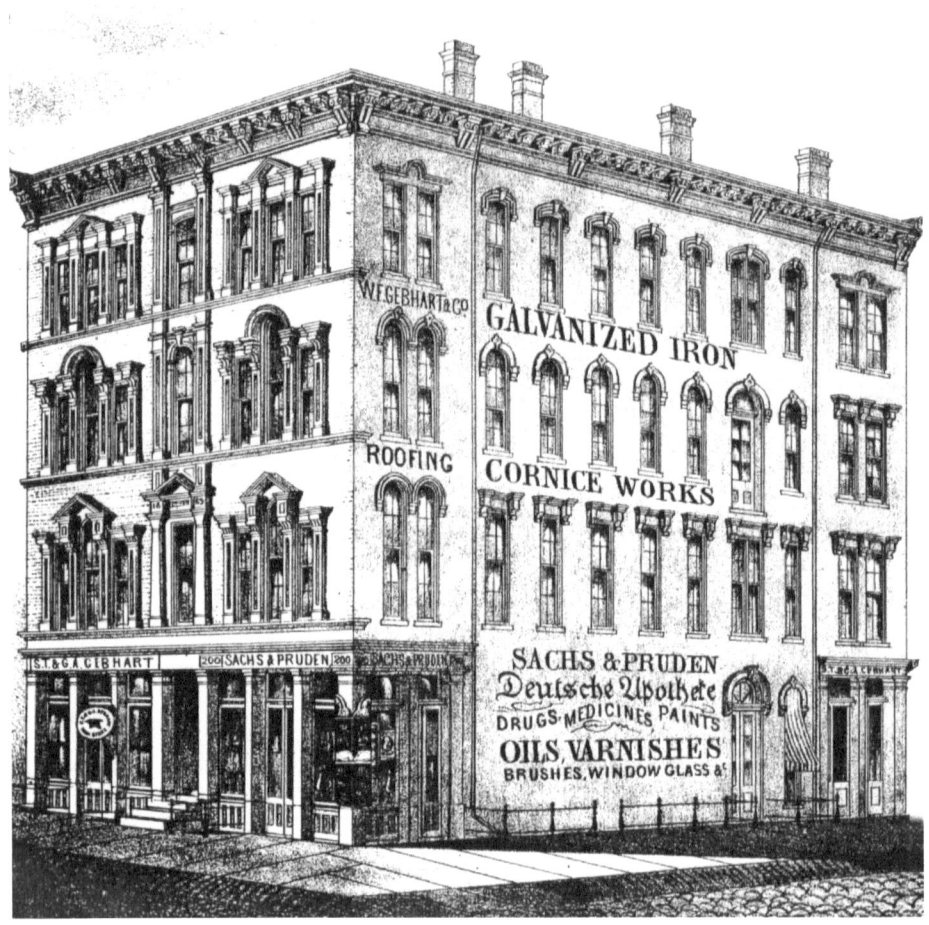

Sachs & Pruden Drug Store was originally located in the Gebhart Building at 200 East Third Street. The drawing shown here is from 1875.

Sachs & Pruden

Edward Sachs and David Pruden owned a drug store at the corner of Third and St. Clair Streets and offered such diverse items as paints, oils, brushes and glass, as well as medicine. In 1883 they opened the Buckeye Bottle Works. Along with ginger ale and flavoring extracts, the two men also manufactured several products with medicinal properties. Their most popular proved to be "A-T-8 Agaric", which was touted as an excellent medicine for the cure of indigestion, dyspepsia and all other diseases of a disordered liver and stomach.

On January 9, 1888 the Sachs-Prudens' Ale Company was incorporated, with the thought of manufacturing ales, beer and other beverages. The two men immediately set out to build a brewery on 79 Wyandot Street. They hired Conrad G. Oland, of Hampshire, England, to supervise its construction. It was four stories tall, 70' x 138' and was thoroughly fireproof, the joists and girders throughout the plant being constructed of steel and the columns of iron. The cellars had a capacity to store 15,000 barrels. The building was completed in September 1888 at a cost of $150,000.

Besides beer, the company also produced "Saline Lemonade", a salty, bitter water that was supposed to aid digestion. A short-lived nostrum, called "Sach's Lithia Water", was pure distilled water to which was added lithium oxide, a strongly alkaline white powder. This type of water was thought to cure, among other things; rheumatic, indigestion, heart disease, insomnia, kidney disease, and headaches.

By 1895 Sachs-Pruden's had gone out of business. Their building on Wyandot was sold to the Dayton Brewing Company, who used it to brew beer. The building currently houses the Hauer Music Company.

Victorian-era trade cards depicting nude women were the exception, rather than the rule. This card was part of a set of four, depicting the four seasons of the year. The insert of the cherub gives the scene a "classical art" look that helps soften the use of a topless woman. Still, Sachs and Pruden probabaly thought that if their "A.-T.-8." wasn't stimulating enough, the card would be.

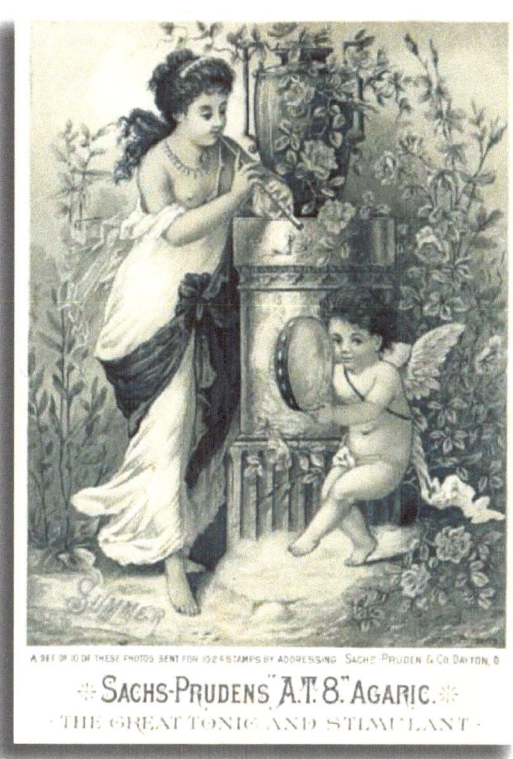

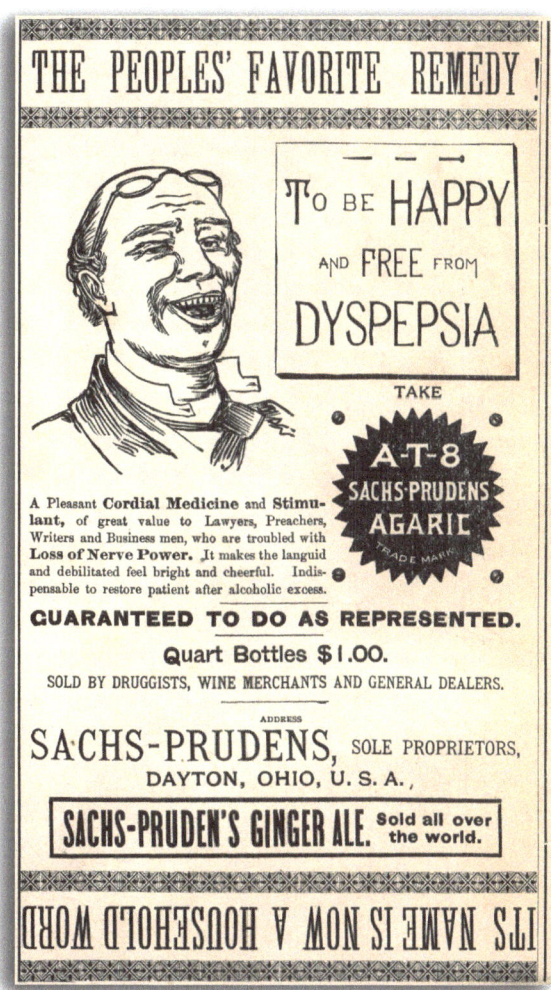

The ingredients of Sachs-Pruden's "A-T-8" are unknown, but it no doubt contained some type of stimulant. The company claimed that the tonic's "actions are immediate, producing at once a feeling of bouyancy to the intellect, removing depression or melancholy (and) contains blood-making, force-generating and life-sustaining properties. And all for the price of one dollar a quart. The man pictured in the ad certainly looks cheerful enough, or perhaps he represents the tonic's claim of being "indispensible to restore patient after alcoholic excess."

The Dr. H. F. Weis Medicine Company

Dr. Henry F. Weis was born in Hesse Darmstadt, Germany in 1832. There he met and married Catherine Kircheimer in 1857. A year later they came to the United States, finally settling at 706 South Wayne Street in 1866. It was there that Dr. Weis would conduct a drug store and practice medicine for nearly half a century.

In 1875 Dr. Weis began selling his "Great Dropsy Remedy." A pint cost $5, a quart was $9, quite costly for this type of medicine at the time.

By 1910 Dr. Weis was offering a plethora of products, including remedies for rheumatism, malaria, piles, and even bed-wetting. His biggest seller was an herb stomach bitter with the unusual name of "Guard on the Rhine." Advertised as a treatment for dyspepsia and other stomach problems, the bitter became so popular that The Dr. H. F. Weis Medicine Company was formed.

There must have been some merit in the different remedies he offered, for Dr. Weis never stopped practicing until his death at the age of 82 in 1915. His wife followed him almost exactly two years later at the age of 83.

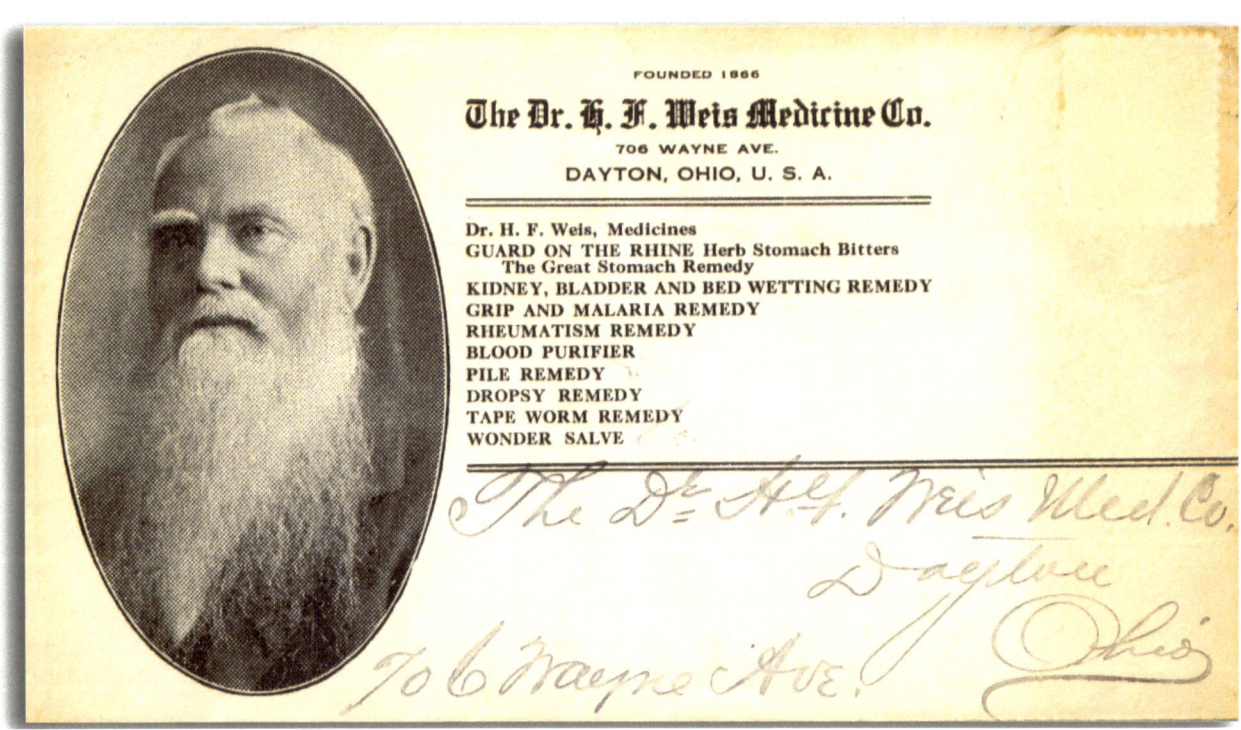

This envelope, used to mail letters and advertisement to various customers, lists the great variety of remedies and other medical offerings manufactured by The Dr. Weis Medicine Company. "Guard on the Rhine" bitters proved so popular that in 1910 the company applied for a trademark on the name, as well as on Dr. Weis' portrait. Both were approved and granted Serial Number 51,912 on September 22, 1910.

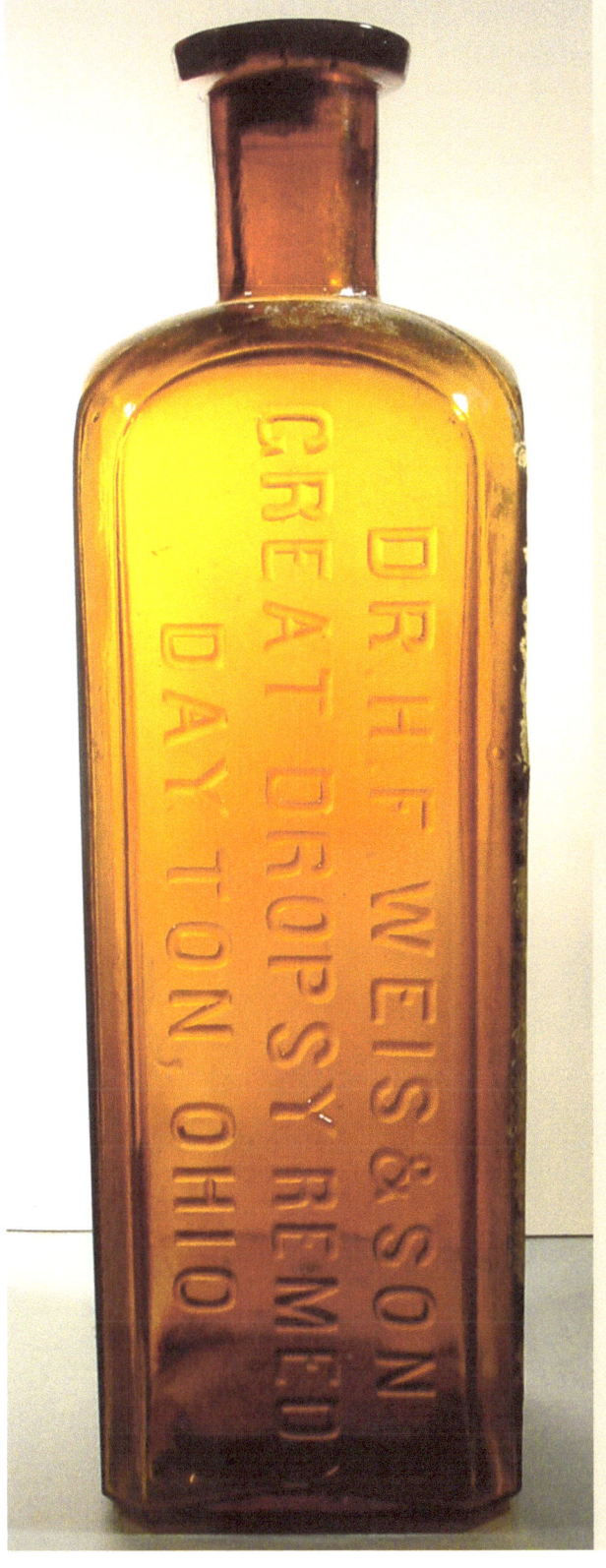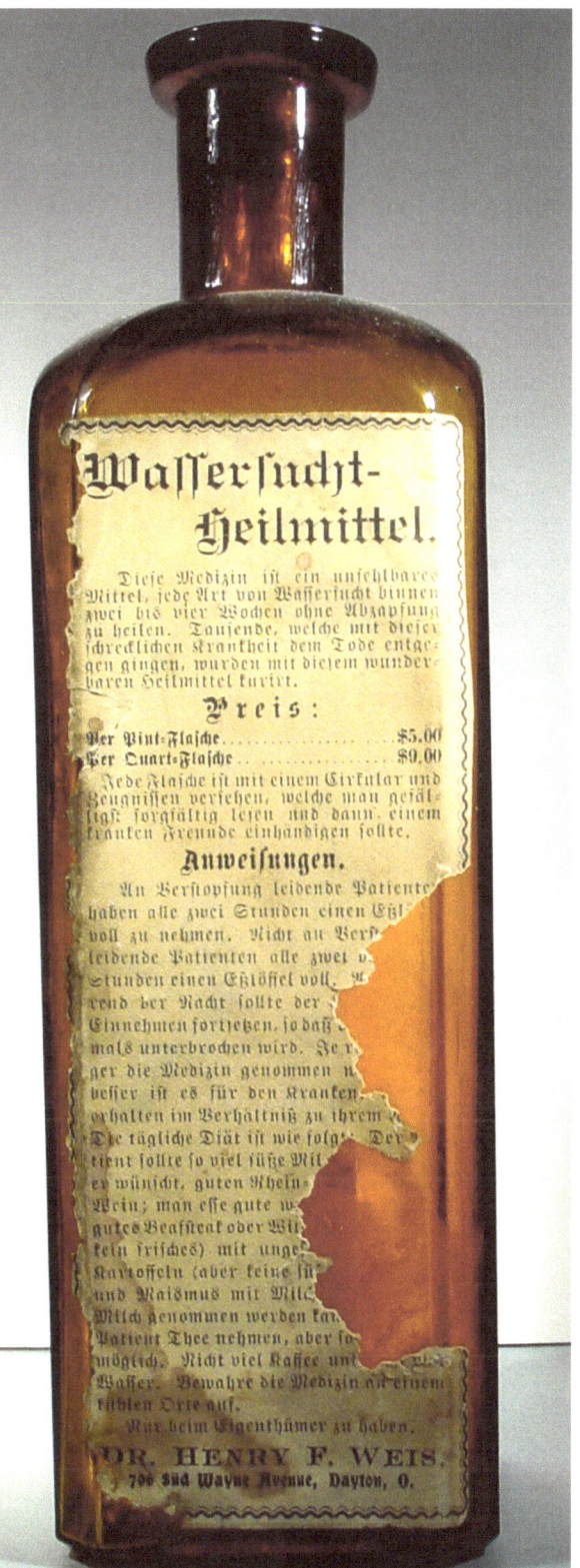

Since almost the very beginning of Dayton's history a vast number of German immigrants chose the Gem City as their final destination. Accordingly, Dr. Weis' offered instructions printed in German on the labels of his "Wassersucht-Heilmittel" or "Dropsy Remedy", while the other side was embossed in English.

Pretzinger's Catarrh Balm

  Although many people have heard of the famous Dayton architect Albert Pretizinger, two of his brothers are also notable. Rudolph and Herman Pretizinger were partners in the drug store business for several decades. Although at first the Pretizinger Bros. drug store sold the usual products, by 1894 the two men had to devote most of their time making their "Pretzinger's Catarrh Balm". Its claim was that, used freely, a diseased or sore spot in the nasal passages would be quickly cured, while graver cases of catarrh or diseases of the head would "yield readily". The Balm became so popular that in 1905 the two brothers formed the Pretizinger Catarrh Balm Co., with Rudolph as president and Herman as Secretary and Treasurer.

  What was Pretzinger's Catarrh Balm made of? The brothers claimed that one of the ingredients was Malay Camphor, grown only on the islands of Borneo and Sumatra in China. Due to its rarity, the special camphor was worth a hundred times more than regular camphor. Very little of it ever found its way to foreign ports, but luckily the Pretzingers had found a steady supplier. Although the Malay Camphor was also mixed with other ingredients, including regular camphors and camphor compounds, the brothers guaranteed that you could smell the "delicate odor" of the Malay Camphor in their preparation. They never claimed that their remedy was a secret - saying it had been used by the Phoenicians, a mysterious, ancient people who developed the modern alphabet over three thousand years ago.

  When Rudolph became ill in 1908 he first took a trip to California, then to Colorado Springs, but when his condition didn't improve, he returned to Dayton. He passed away February 14, 1909 and was buried at Woodland. His brother continued to sell the balm until 1922. Several sources state that a product named "Pretzinger's Nasal Balm" was selling as late as 1948, but no other information on this is known.

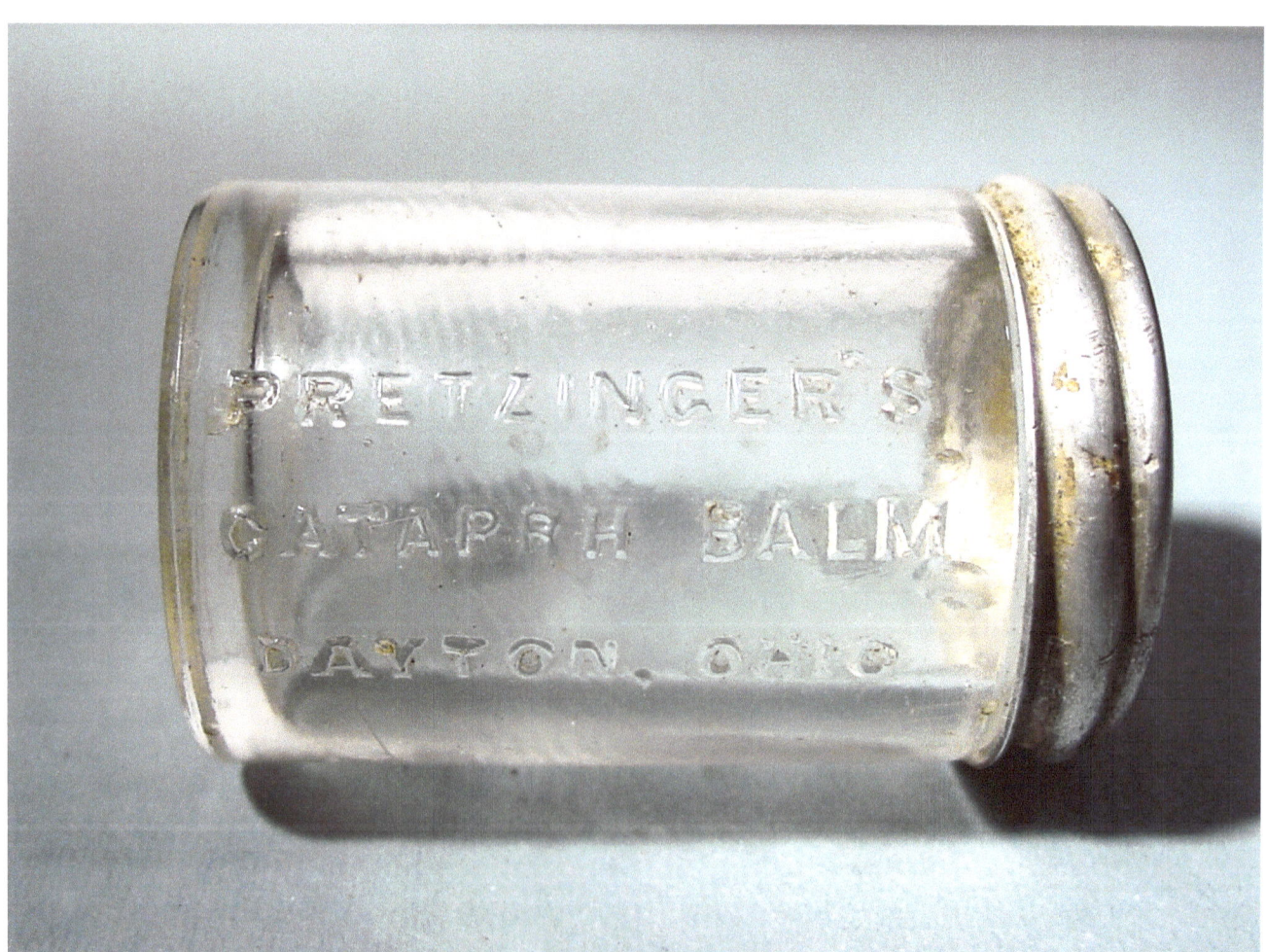

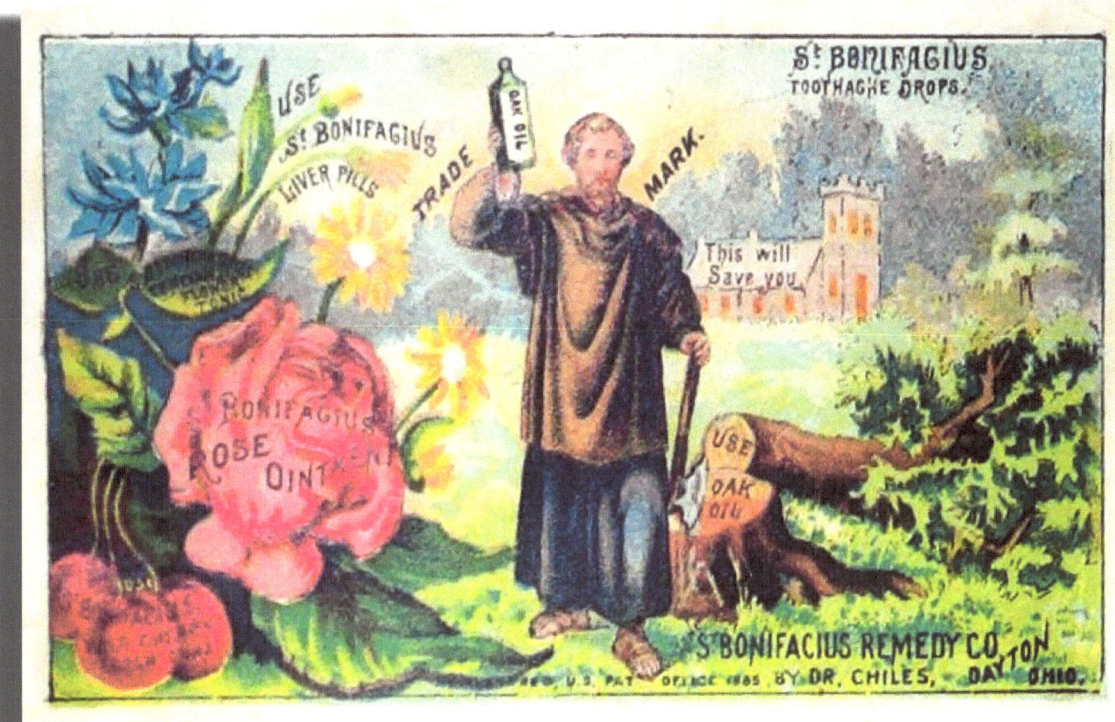

St. Bonifacius Gentian Flower Tonic

Dr. J. W. Chiles was a versatile man, to say the least. In 1882 he began advertising himself as a "Veterinary Druggist and Chemist" who sold a varitey of remedies "meant for horses, cattle, pigs, sheep and poultry, also for the diseases of the human body." In 1885 Dr. Chiles registered the name "St. Bonifacius Remedy Company" and began offering remedies of his own making, including "St. Bonifacius Tootache Drops", "Wild Cherry Cough Cure", "Liver Pill", "Rose Ointment" and "Oak Oil".

The main remedy sold by the company seemed to be "St. Bonifacius Gentian Flower Tonic". The tonic was advertsied as being far superior to any other tonic in use for the cure of scrofula (a tuberculosis tumor of the neck) and as a blood purifier.

In 1886 Dr. Chiles closed his shop and left Dayton.

It should be noted that St. Marculf, not St. Bonifacius, is the best-known patron saint of scrofulous diseases. After touching his relics, French kings were reported to be able to cure scrofula.

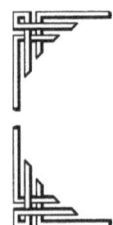
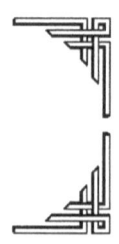

Chapter Eight
Back to Nature

It was the medical profession itself that helped strengthen the idea that the more modern medicines sometimes hurt more than they cured. As doctors began to suggest that the use of mercury, lead, arsenic and morphine were inherently dangerous, people wondered what other ingredients might be contained in their prescriptions that could harm them. The idea behind a "natural" product appealed to those who wanted to hark back to a simpler time, when unadulterated plants and herbs were used for safer and purer remedies.

The use of herbs for medicinal purposes have been used by man for centuries. But the patent medicine companies carried it to extreme, promising cures that no one root or bark of a tree could deliver. Natural remedies often contained a large number of herbs, with the hope that at least one of the ingredients would work its magic on whatever ailment the buyer might have.

Although best know for his "Wine of Tar", Dr. Oliver Crook also manufactured several other herbal medicines over the years. Dr. Crook's "Vegetable Extract" was for use on tumors, old sores, chronic diseases of the eyes and all diseases which supposedly arose from impurities of the blood. Ads prclaimed that it was purely vegetable and contained no opium.

The best way of getting rid of a cough or cold, according to Dr. Crook, was to buy a bottle of his "Benzoin Elixir". In order to make the medicine, deep cuts had to be made into the bark of Siam and Sumatra Benzoin trees. Under the shock the trees would discharge a yellowish-brown liquid. This was the benzoin. When it was sufficiently hard enough, the collectors would peel it off with their tools, which would then be mixed wth other secret ingredients. The elixir was also good for relieving all bronchial troubles and had never been known to fail when used for croup. Sales must have been slow, however, as it was only available from 1861 to 1866.

Dr. Crook claimed that his Vegetable Extract cured cancer, while his Benzoin Elixir cured "bleeding of the lungs", a sure sign of consumption. Neither worked.

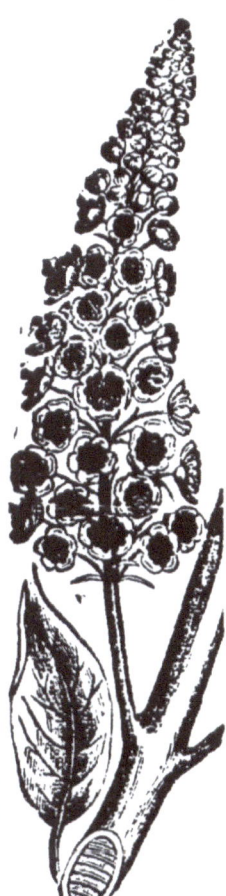
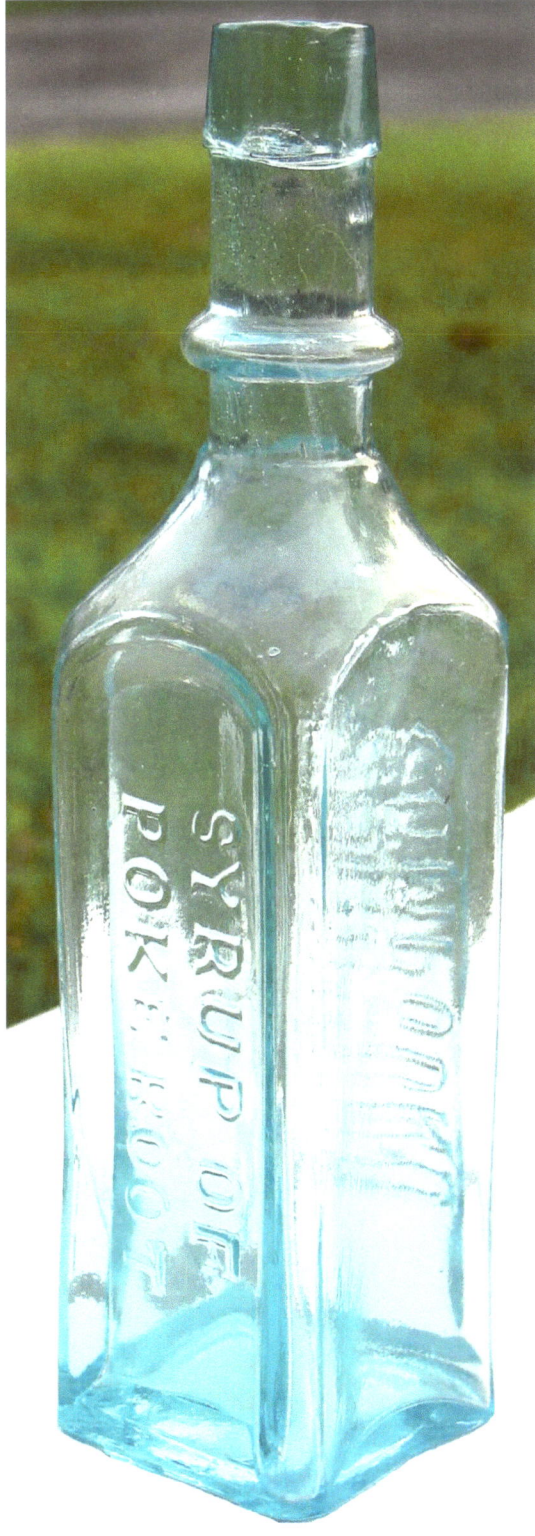

For centuries the poke root plant had a reputation for curing rheumatism. In 1871, after twenty-five years of hard work, Dr. Oliver Crook had finally perfected his "Compound Syrup of Poke Root" so that it also cured chronic diseases of ANY kind, including diseases of the skin, eruptions, pimples, boils, ring-worm, sores, diseases of the eyes, pains in the bones and even "broken-down constitutions".

Hirsch's Sarsparilla

Albert A. Hirsch was one of the more successful smaller dealers in medicines in Dayton. In 1895, when he was only 21 years old, Albert began manufacturing medicines out of his home. He would continue to do so for the next forty-one years. One of the many products Albert had to offer was a potion called "Hirsch's Sarsaparilla", which helped those who suffered from rheumatism. Not to be confused with root beer, sarsaparilla was first used as a cure for syphilis four hundred years ago, then eventually became known to help ease the pain of arthritis and heal ulcers. In 1960 the Food and Drug Administration banned sassafras root and bark as food after they were discovered to contain large amounts of safrole, a chemical that causes cancer and liver damage. Commercial root beer still tastes like sassafras because the FDA allows the use of a "sassafras extract," from which the safrole has been carefully removed. Sassafras is so versatile and so effective that even today it's used in certain medicine.

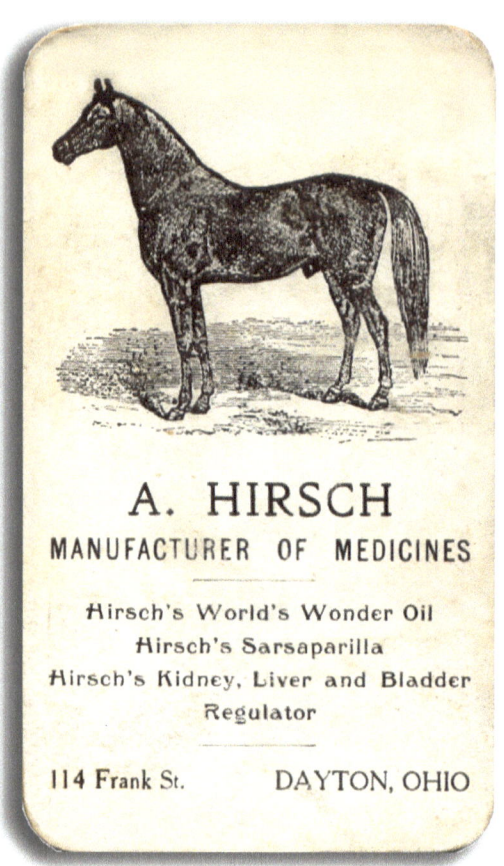

Ra-Mo-Na Herbs Tablets

In 1915 the Ramona Herb Company introduced Ra-Mo-Na Herbs Tablets. Each tablet was made of eight different herbs, roots and barks that worked together to naturally cleanse the system and "assist the various organs to perform their functions in Natures own way." In case this sounded as if the tablet was merely a laxative, the company made it clear that the herbs effectively cured stomach trouble, corrected the liver and helped those with weak kidneys. It was popular enough in nearby cities, but never took off nationally. Business eventually slacked off and the Ramona Herb Company had closed its doors by 1922.

Tona Vita

In 1911 The Approved Formula Company introduced a superb tonic called "Tona Vita". Nationally advertised as "bottled rest", the company appealed to customers who had been "beaten down by life."

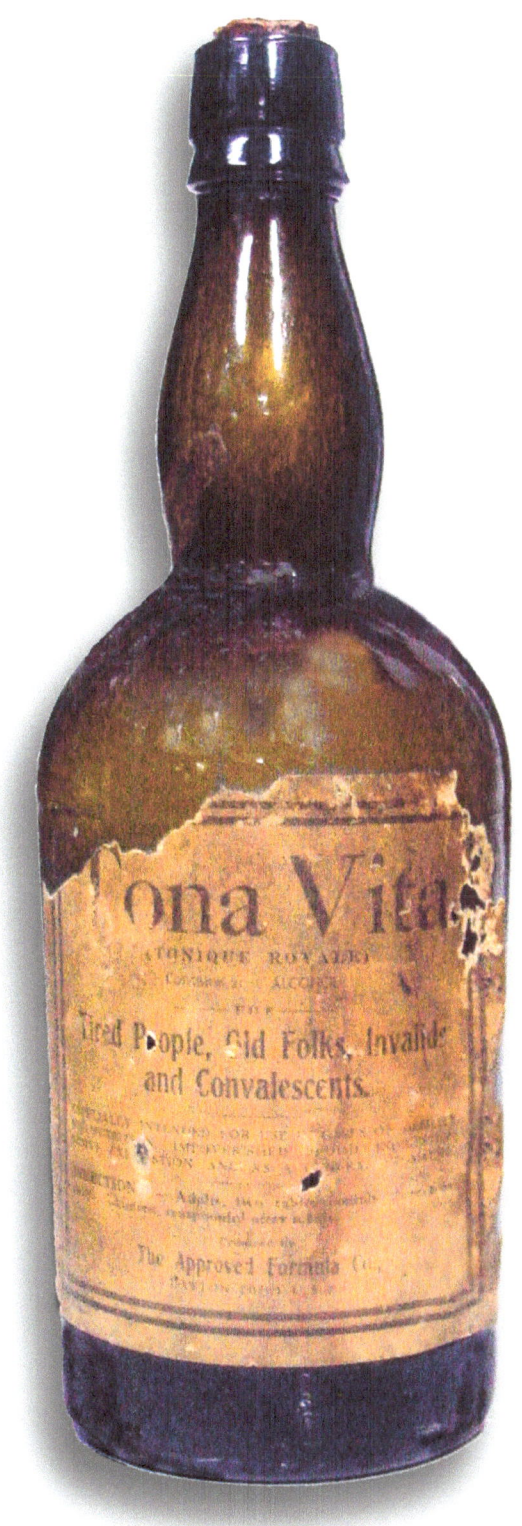

When people of wealth become debilitated and run down in health they go to high priced sanitariums and health resorts to be built up again. But what about the thousands of debilitated nervous men and women, with no vitality or ambition, who have neither the time nor money to spare for such luxuries as sanitariums? If you are debilitated and run down, don't allow this miserable condition to last a day longer. Let Tona Vita build you up and bring you back to health.

Making people fear that they could be sick without even knowing it was a sure way of selling nostrums and The Approved Formula Company were experts at cultivating that fear. A "specialist" was quoted in the Indianapolis Star as saying it was possible that nearly every family in Indianapolis was suffering from an attack of nervous debility.

The public do not realize what a tremendous number of people among those who live in the larger cities like Indianapolis are afflicted with this modern plague in a more or less aggravated form. Most of the so-called kidney trouble, nearly all indigestion and fully half the headaches in Indianapolis can be attributed solely to nervous debility, superinduced by the strain of modern city life.

But, fortunately, Tona Vita was guaranteed to cure the constant sufferer from stomach ailments, headaches and other troubles caused by stress.

From time to time the Connecticut Agricultural Experiment Station in New Haven, Connecticut would analyze various proprietary medicines that were found advertised in their local newspapers. On October 10, 1916, the New Haven Department of Health published the Station's findings. One of those products happened to be Tona Vita. They found Tona Vita to be a sherry wine that had been slightly flavored with meat extract and quite useless for what it was being advertised for. However, since the tonic had nearly a 21% alcohol content, it might just have been the kind of pick-me-up a fellow needed at the end of a long day.

Perhaps the bad publicity hurt sales or maybe it had already run its course, but either way Tona Vita was off the market a short time later.

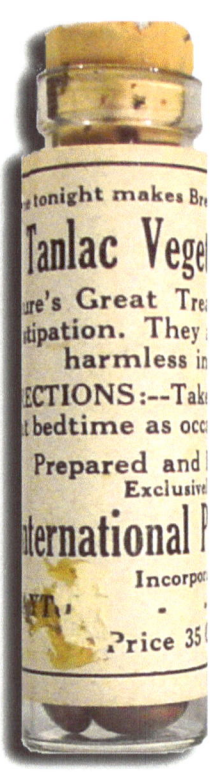

Tanlac Vegetable Pills

Tanlac Vegetable Pills were made by the Cooper Medicine Company. The pills were to be taken in conjunction with the company's Tanlac Tonic in order to cleanse the body of impurities. Advertised as "Nature's Treatment for Constipation", the all-vegetable pills helped eliminate headaches, indigestion, sour stomach, bad breath and even pimples that were supposedly caused whenever one's "system is clogged up with waste products" as the ads delicately put it. Sufferers were directed to take two tablets at first, then another each night until they were "regular" again. As fiber really is a good way to ease constipation, it is in all likelihood that these little pills actually worked. When International Proprietaries took over the Cooper Medicine Company, they continued to offer the product as "an essential and vitally important part of the Tanlac Treatment".

Botanic Lung Syrup

Not much is known about the Botanic Remedy Company, except for the fact that they offered a bottled remedy for asthma and consumption called "Botanic Lung Syrup". Before modern pharmacy, physicians were trained in botany and spent time collecting and studying American flora and the medicinal uses of plants. The word Botanic immediately let the buyers of this "Lung Syrup" know that the tonic had been extracted from plants. The statement that it had been prepared from an ancient German formula would also have been a comfort to the many Daytonians who were from that country.

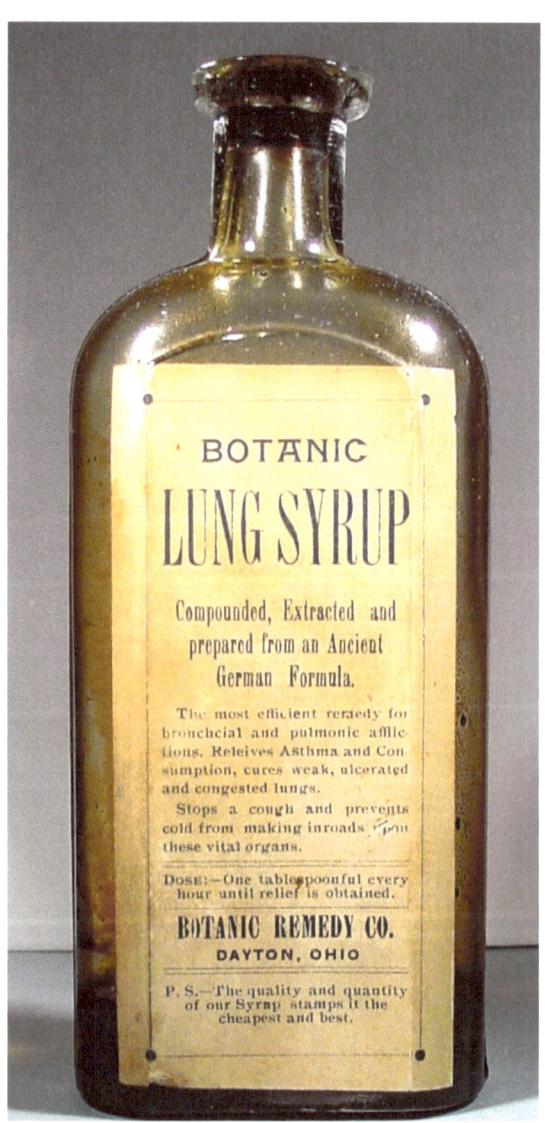

Pepgen

The American Drug Company opened on the 4th floor at 24 North Jefferson Street in 1918 and began offering three products to help relieve mankind from its pain and suffering. Pepgen Liniment, which contained mustard, red pepper, sassafras, menthol and ammonia, was applied to the skin to ease the aches of lumbago, neuralgia, and sprains. It could also be taken internally for coughs, colds or cramps. Pepgen Laxative Tablets were meant to assist those who suffered from constipation and an inactive liver. But the big seller was Pepgen Tonic.

Pepgen Tonic was touted as a "delightful appetizer and general invigorant". Due to the Pure Food and Drugs Act the company was careful not to claim that its tonic cured anything. Instead, it allowed the public to make these claims for them. D. J. O'Donnell, publisher of the *Montgomery Reporter* newspaper, in Dayton, wrote of how the tonic gave him back his strength and made him a new man. John Hatcher, of Decatur, Illinois, suffered with dyspepsia for two years before trying the medicine. After taking Pepgen he was quoted as saying, "I feel 'bully' now." Soon scores of citizens were declaring relief from long-standing cases of stomach, kidney and liver troubles.

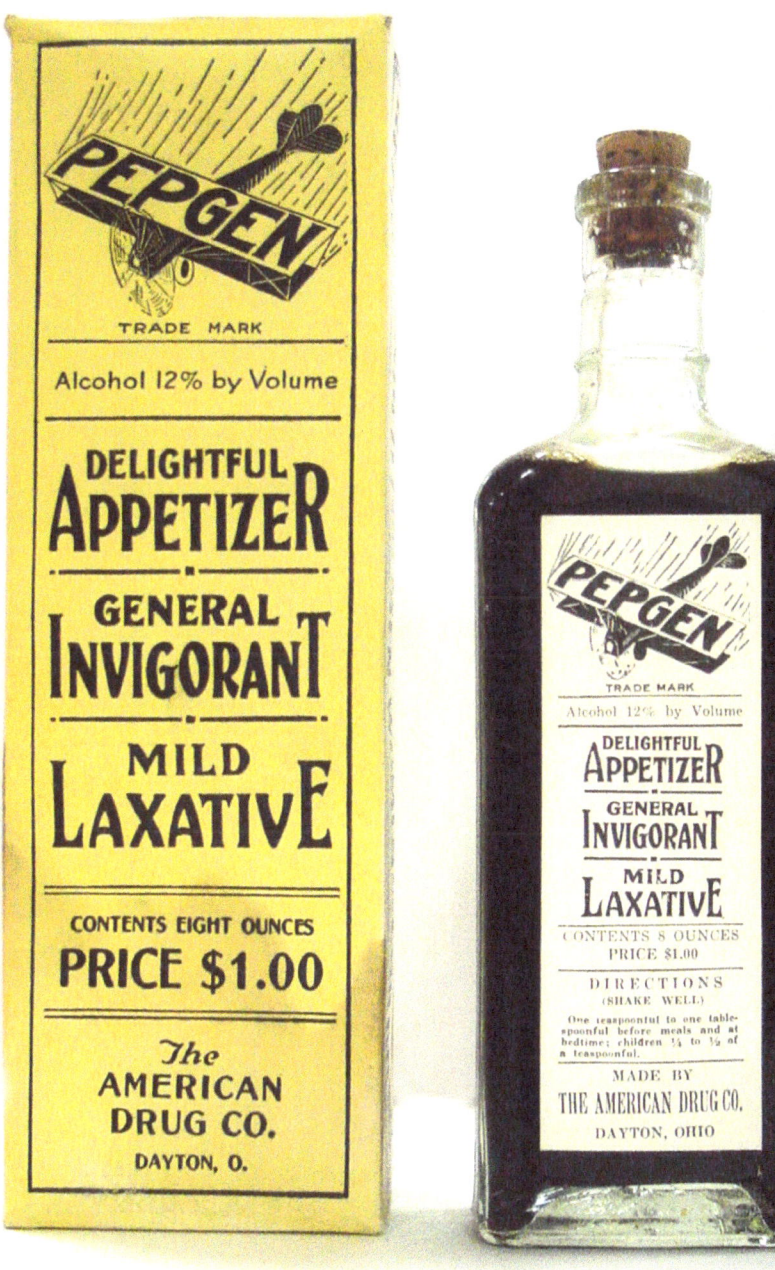

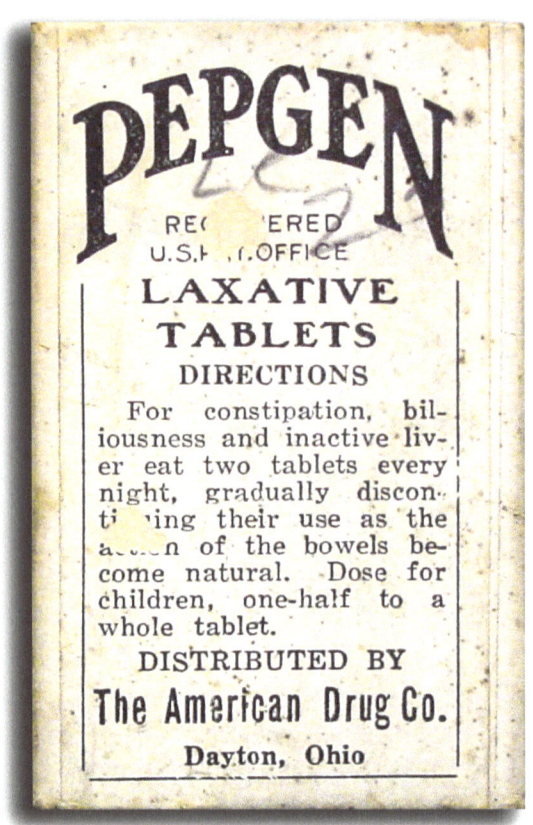

relieved pain and plaintain leaves operated on the nerves to sooth them and induce sleep. Peruvian Bark, which was considered one of the greatest stomach and liver medicines ever discovered, was an especially important ingredient. Oddly, the article actually emphasized the fact that the Peruvian Bark had been prepared without alcohol, yet the Pepgen Tonic had an alcohol content of 12%.

The American Drug Company was no longer listed in the Dayton city directory after 1922. The Burge-Layton Company, of Dayton, went on to manufacture the tonic. Pepgen could still be found in drug stores in Indiana and Ohio through the early 1930s.

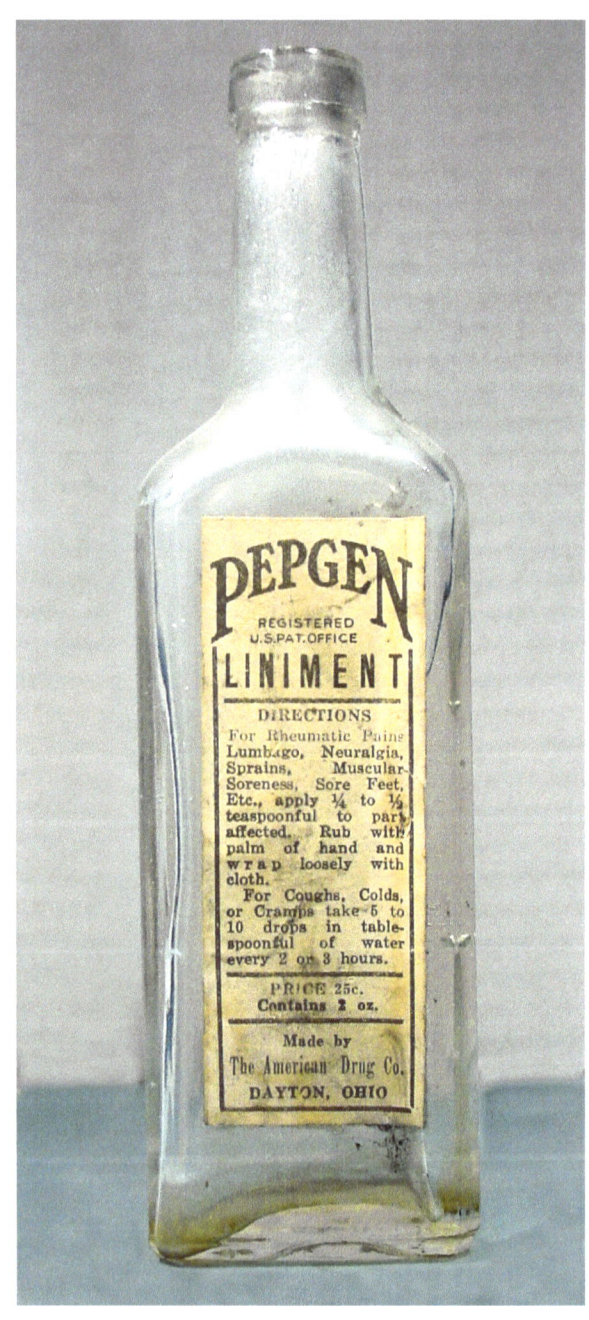

The company stated that W. R. Cooper, a scientist from Dayton, was largely responsible for the discovery of the Pepgen tonic. He had worked with a number of expert chemists for over three years before finally perfecting the seventeen ingredients of herbs, barks, roots and flowers that made up the natural remedy. Although it is hard to be positively sure, it is very likely that W. R. Cooper was, in fact, William R. Cooper, brother of Lee T. Cooper, of the Cooper Medicine Company.

In 1919 a headline in the local newspapers caught the public's attention. Capital letters in bold print read "WILL PAY $1,000.00 REWARD". The substance of the following text more or less turned out to be an ad for Pepgen. The American Drug Company stated it had been rumored that people were being paid for their testimonials to endorse worthless medicine. The company stressed that they had never practiced that sort of deception and were willing to pay $1,000 if anyone could prove they had. Readers of the article were then regaled with a long description of what ingredients the medicine contained and why they had been included. Gentian root was added to aid digestion, fringe tree bark exerted an influence on the liver, blach cohosh effected the muscular system and

Chapter Nine
Indian Medicines

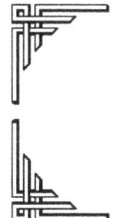
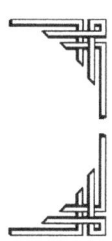

Explorers of the New World found themselves in a land quite different from the country they had left behind. They depended, to some extent, on imports from the Old World; but sometimes supplies were cut off due to war or other factors. They soon noticed that Native Americans utilized healing plants of the forests and prairies to make salves and poultices for their ills. Many of these herbal cures soon found their way into the white physician's medicine bag.

Nicholaes van Wassenaer, a Dutch colonist, observed that the Indians he encountered were in exceptionally good health.

There are few or none cross-eyed, blind, crippled, lame, hunch-backed, or limping men; all are well-fashioned people, strong and sound of body, well-fed, without blemish.

In 1894, Dr. J. L. Neave reported in the *Cincinnati Medical Journal* of how enamored people were with the secret mixture of roots, berries and herbs that the Indians used to naturally heal themselves.

The American Indian has been, and is given credit for a wonderful knowledge of medicine. Compounds purporting to have originated among some of the numerous tribes, have attributed to them wonderful healing powers, and are readily sold to persons at good prices; who would not be guilty of paying a like amount to their local physician, for real services rendered in the past. They will pay the Indian Doctor, or the man who sells Indian cures, a good round sum for the article vended, and never question but that they have value received.

Others eventually began to notice and soon Native American cures became very popular. Some doctors began advertising as being of this persuasion, and patent medicine men were quick to pick up on the idea themselves. The American Indian was probably the most used symbol for these natural remedies. By the turn of the century a somewhat romantic view of the Wild West had taken hold. Colorful chiefs and beautiful Indian maidens became the symbols associated with this type of medicine. The stories of how the nostrum sellers were let in on the generations-old secret medicines varied, but many dealt with how the nostrum seller somehow saved the life of a medicine man or chief of a certain tribe. The Indian whose life was saved would show his gratitude by sharing the secret ingredients of a medicine passed down through the generations which were sure to cure whatever disease might be in vouge at the time. Books such as the popular *The North American Indian Doctor, or Nature's Method of Curing and Preventing Disease According to the Indians* were soon quite popular. After all, who could argue with the brilliant advertiser who asked "whoever saw a sick Indian?" Forget the fact that most people had never seen an Indian at all, sick or not. Customers were interested in buying these native remedies and Dayton nostrum manufacturers were more than happy to accommodate them.

J. Foley's Indian Botanic Balsam

John Foley was born in Boston, Massachusetts in 1807. He and his wife, Abigail, are first listed in the Dayton city directory in 1858. John gave his occupation as a manufacturer of "J. Foley's Indian Botanic Balsam" which he made and sold out of his home at the southeast corner of Third and Ringold Street. In 1862 he moved the place of business to 25 Terry Street and still later to 5 Clinton Street. Although he was never listed as a physician in any Dayton directories, in the 1870 census John gave his occupation as a "Botanic Physician." This term was used by doctors whose medicines consisted mainly of roots and herbs.

Although his Balsam never made it to the big-time, it did rate several ads in the Lorain County Eagle newspaper. The ad stated that Foley's nostrum was the best medicine in use for the lungs and that it was for sale by T. Potter at Room #4 in the Beebe Block in Elyria, Ohio.

In 1875 Foley applied for, and was granted, two trademarks for his medicines. Patent Trademark #2,864 was described as having the words "Foley's Indian Botanic Balsam For The Lungs" arranged above and below a drawing of a landscape. In the foreground was the figure of an Indian standing upon the banks of a stream, holding in his right hand a bow, and in his left, partly extended, a bundle of herbs. On the opposite bank of the stream, which was covered with trees, stood two deer at the water's edge, drinking.

Patent Trademark #2,865 was described as having a landscape with the figures of two Indians upon the bank of a stream. The one on the left was kneeling on a rock under a tree and leveling his gun at a deer in the distance. The Indian to the right had in his right hand a bow and in his left a bundle of herbs, representing the balsam used in the medicine mixture. On the farther bank of the stream was a thick forest. Over the border of the picture the sun was rising and in the divergent rays was the word "Foley's." Just under the picture were the words "Indian Botanic Balsam." It is unknown if these trademarks were ever used.

John Foley died two years later and was buried at Woodland Cemetery on September 1, 1877.

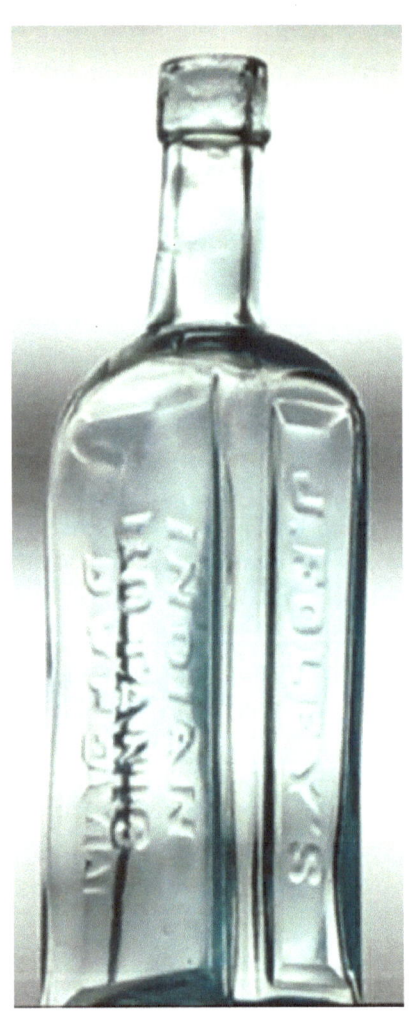
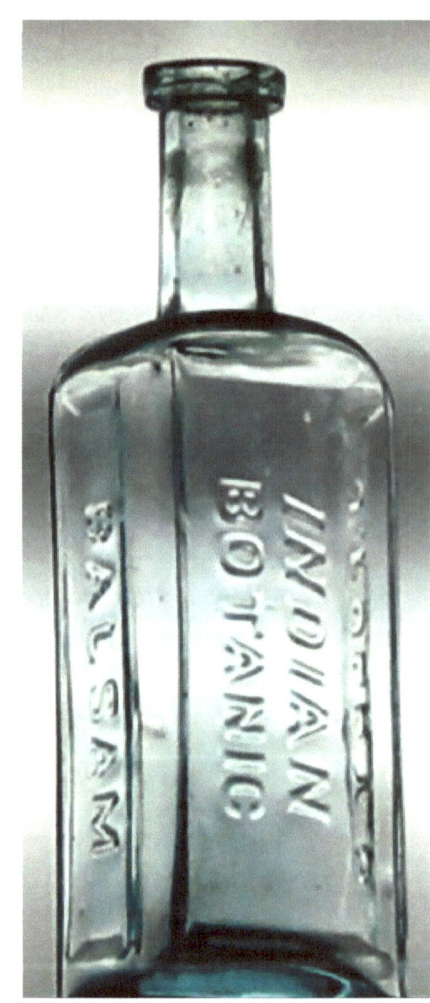

Two variations of the bottles Foley used to sell his Indian Botanic Balsam. Balsam was used by some to try and cure lung affections. The balsam was thought to lubricate the bronchial tubes and air sacs, remove inflammation and assist the lungs in throwing off disease. This was supposedly especially helpful to those who suffered from consumption. Upon the first indication of a cold in the head or throat, the user was to rub the ointment around the throat and over the chest. This would prevent the cold from entering the lungs. It was said that those who suffered from consumption were also curable, but these patients might have to use the medication for the rest of their lives.

Redfern's Indian Tonic

Edgar S. Gebhart started the Redfern Medicine Company in 1927. It's sole product was Redfern's Indian Tonic, a potion that worked miracles in relieving indigestion, heartburn, nausea and a sour stomach. It also helped calm ruffled nerves.

The story behind the recipe for the wonderful tonic is that it was obtained in 1796 by Robert Redfern from the Miami Indians, who once inhabited the territory now embracing Dayton and southwestern Ohio. In case this sounded too primitive, the manufacturer added that the product had since been "improved by more modern medical discoveries. The principal ingredients of the formula consisted of juice from the papaw, golden seal, pepsin and malt, as well as a liberal dose of alcohol, 18% to be exact. The funny thing was, Gebhart's home and business was located at 1048 Redfern Avenue, which was probably just a coincidence. Gebhart's business eventually grew sour and closed in 1933.

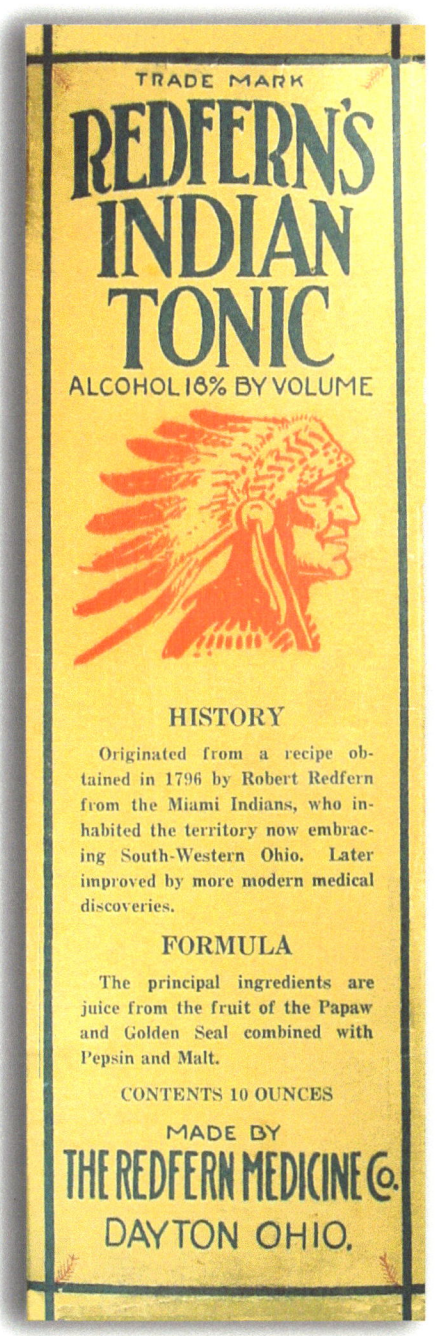
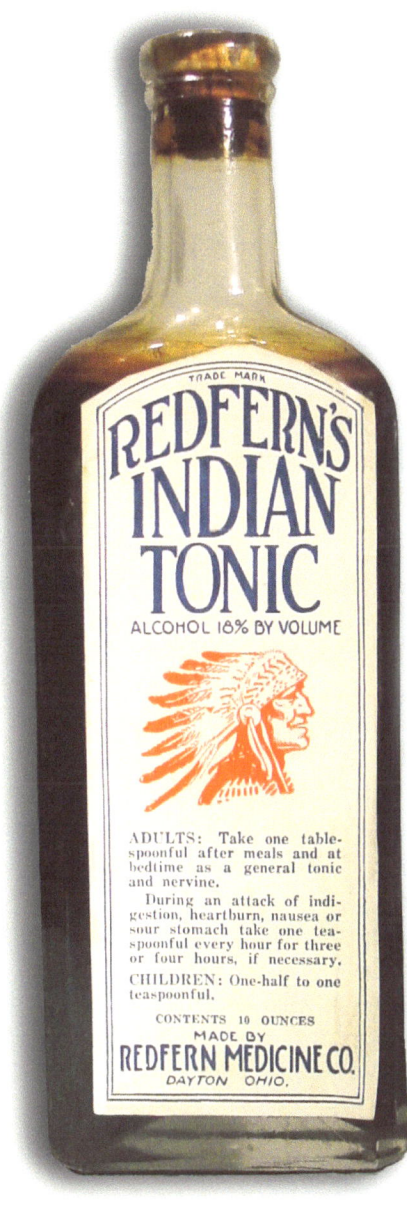

Ki-A-Wah

The Indian Medicine Company opened in 1904 at 303 West Third Street and began selling Ki-A-Wah, a medicine good for many "cures" according to its advertisements. Users of the tonic stated in strong terms that Ki-A-Wah was a valuable medicine. After using less than one bottle, H. J. Williams, of Middletown, claimed to be completely cured his stomach troubles and wouldn't take $1,000 for the good it had done him. And this was a time when $1000 was a bunch of money. Daytonian J. N. Johnson had a bad case of kidney and bladder trouble and his wife was so twisted up by rheumatism that she could no longer walk or use her hands. A half-dozen bottles of Ki-A-Wah later and both had been completely cured of their troubles. Business must have been good at first, for the following year the Indian Medicine Company was incorporated and moved to the southwest corner of Concord and Cincinnati streets. Elwood E. Rice, who had previously been a grain dealer, was president of the company.

The Ki-A-Wah medicine, good as it supposedly was, only made it into a few drug stores. The Indian Medicine Company folded in 1906, perhaps under pressure of the new Pure Food and Drugs Act. Elwood Rice went on to open the R. & R. Sign Company the following year.

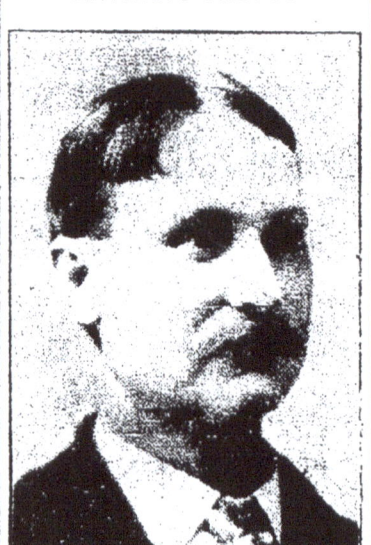

KI-A-WAH'S FRIENDS.

MR. J. J. WILLIAMS CERTAINLY THINKS KI-A-WAH A VALUABLE MEDICINE.
Indian Medicine Co., Dayton, O.
Gentlemen:—I have been troubled with stomach trouble and indigestion for over a year and have doctored with two doctors who, I am confident, did their best to help me, but couldn't do me a penny's worth of good. I have taken less than one bottle of your Ki-A-Wah, and it has entirely cured me. It is certainly a positive cure for stomach trouble and I am pleased to recommend it as such. I wouldn't take $1,000 for the good it has done me.
H. J. WILLIAMS,
119 E. 3rd St.
Middletown, O.

Indian Herb Tablets

George H. Parker began as an agent for the Great American Herb Company in 1911. Soon George was manufacturing "Indian Herb Tablets" which he recommended the user take for a variety of ailments, including constipation, rheumatism and catarrh. George's son, Charles, joined his father in 1919, before taking over the business in 1923. With the help of sales of "Parker's K. & P. Pink Herb Tablets" which were to be used to regulate and purify the kidneys, the company was able to stay in business until 1938.

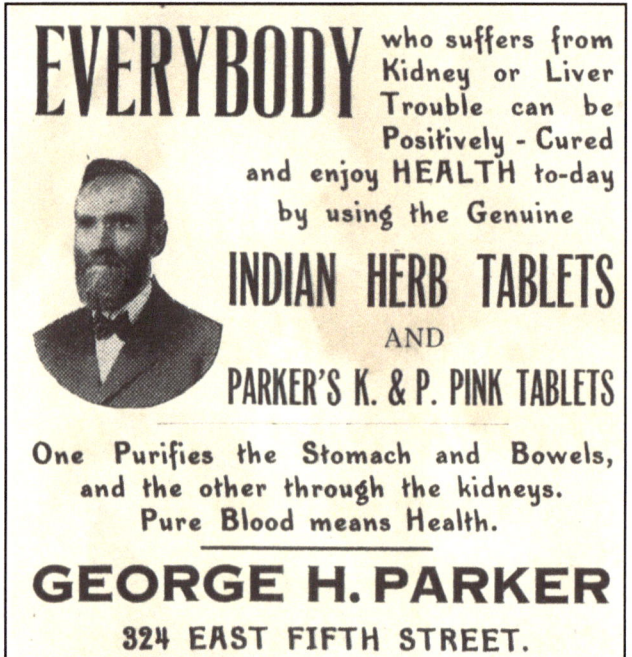

Great Indian Asthma & Hay Fever Remedy

G. W. Shade & Co. began offering the "Great Indian Asthma and Hay Fever Remedy and Indian Tonic" in 1909. The company bragged that their remedy was "the only absolute cure known for asthma and hay fever. In 1927 it became the Shade Medicine Co. The company closed in 1938.

SHADE G. W. & CO.,
(G. W. S. & S. A. Shade) Manufacturers of the Great Indian Asthma and Hay Fever Remedy and Indian Tonic. The only absolute cure known, made purely of Roots and Herbs, 823 N Main; Telephones Bell 2035

Chapter Ten
Miscellaneous Nostrums

Harter's Little Liver Pills

Although better known for their "Iron Tonic" the Dr. Harter Medicine Company also widely advertised "Harter's Little Liver Pills". One of its many uses was to relieve sick headaches by assisting the liver in cleansing the blood of bile. The company chose an unusual form of advertising to get its message across.

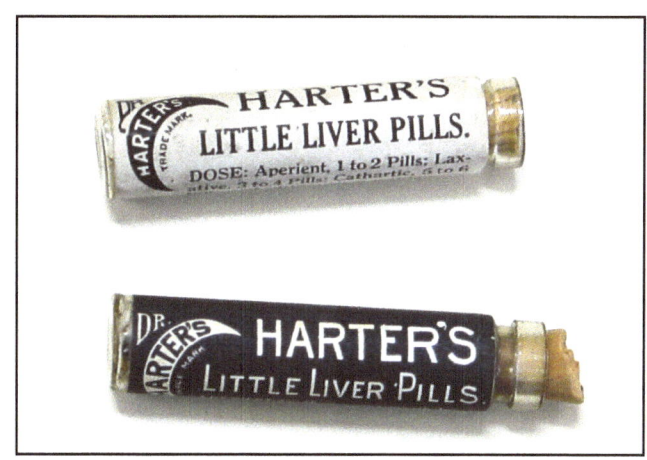

Your Head Aches, does it? Well, don't blame us. We are not responsible for your ignorance of mental and physical wants… You are blind to your own interest when you neglect to heed nature's warning with a reliable remedy within your reach at a trifling expense.

Such abuse must have worked, for the Little Liver Pills became one of the company's best sellers. And, you ask, which came first, "Harter's Little Liver Pills" or "Carter's Little Liver Pills"? Dr. Harter seems to have introduced his liver pills sometime in the 1860s. Since the Carter Medicine Company wasn't founded until 1880, then Dr. Harter wins the battle. But the Carter Medicine Company wins the war, since it is still in business and still sells its pills under the name of "Carter's Laxative".

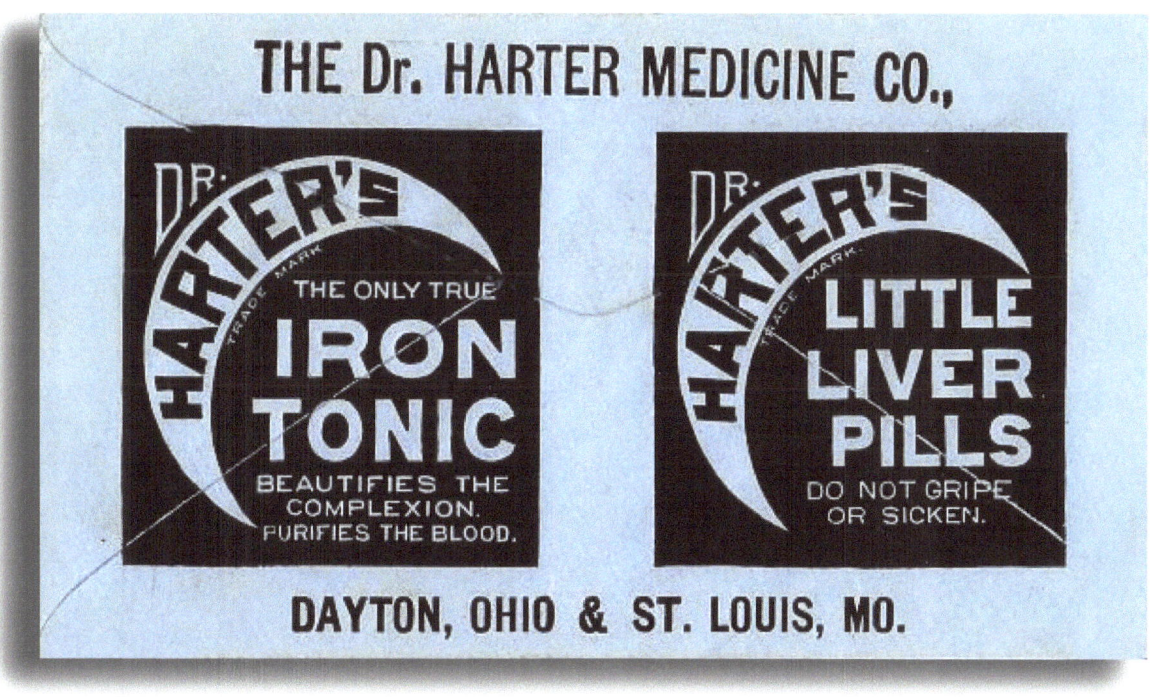

Arras' Celebrated Remedies

Sometime around 1870 Nicholas Arras left his job as a day laborer and began peddling medicines his wife, Ann, created at home. Ann's self-made remedies were sure to cure, among other things, cholera and cholera morbus, asthma, croup and neuralgia. She also had on hand "Eye Water, a Certain Cure of Sore Eyes", toothache and headache powders, plaster for bunions and ointment for wounds. Mrs. Arras' remedies could be obtained at her office, which was also her residence, at 5 Webster Street. The couple later moved to 39 South Van Lear Street in 1884. Ann continued to sell her remedies until 1891.

Mrs. A. E. Arras' CELEBRATED REMEDIES
FOR THE CURE OF
Griping Pains, Diarrhœa, Colic, Cholera and Cholera Morbus, Croup, Asthma, Bronchitis, Neuralgia, Toothache and Headache.

Neutralizing Powders, for Infants and Adults. Eye Water, a Certain Cure for Sore Eyes. Also, Anti-Bilious Pills, Plaster for Bunions and Corns, and Ointment for Burns, Scalds and Wounds. Also, other valuable Medicines always on hand.

☞ These celebrated articles for the sure relief of those suffering from the above-named diseases, can be obtained of Mrs. Arras at her residence,

No. 5 Webster Street, bet. First and Second, **DAYTON, OHIO.**

Concentrated Oil of Pine Compound

In 1908 the Globe Pharmaceutical Company began running ads across the country for their product "Concentrated Oil of Pine Compound." Readers were given a recipe using the compound that was guaranteed to "Break up a cold in 24 hours or cure any cough that is curable." The recipe called for a half-pint of whiskey, two ounces of glycerine and one-half ounce of "Concentrated Oil of Pine" to be mixed together. The resulting liquid was to be taken in doses of a teaspoon to a tablespoon every four hours. The concentrate was sold in one-half ounce vials. Readers were warned not to use imitations as they could "work havoc to the kidneys" and were assured that the compound put out by Globe Pharmaceutical was guaranteed under the Pure Food and Drugs Act.

A short time later the company found themselves under attack by that very same government agency. A sample of the pine preparation had been analyzed by the Bureau of Chemistry and found more or less to be turpentine. The findings were that "the composition did not in any way warrant the use of the name 'Concentrated Oil of Pine Compound,' and the statement that it was such was false, misleading and deceptive." The Globe Pharmaceutical Company, in the persons of William E. Pilkington and A. P Foose, pleaded guilty to the charge of misbranding and paid a fine and the costs of the prosecution.

HOME RECIPE FOR COLDS.

Will Break Up a Cold In 24 Hours or Cure Any Cough That Is Curable.

Mix half pint of good whisky with two ounces of glycerine and add one-half ounce Concentrated oil of pine. The bottle is to be well shaken each time and used in doses of a teaspoonful to a tablespoonful every four hours. The Concentrated oil of pine comes in one-half ounce vials packed securely in tin screw top cases which are intended to protect it from light and retain all the original ozone. It is a product of the laboratories of the Globe Pharmaceutical Co, of Dayton, Ohio, and is guaranteed under the National Pure Food and Drug Act. Don't use bulk oil of pine or imitations of Concentrated. They are insoluble and work havoc to the kidneys Any druggist has the Concentrated oil of pine.

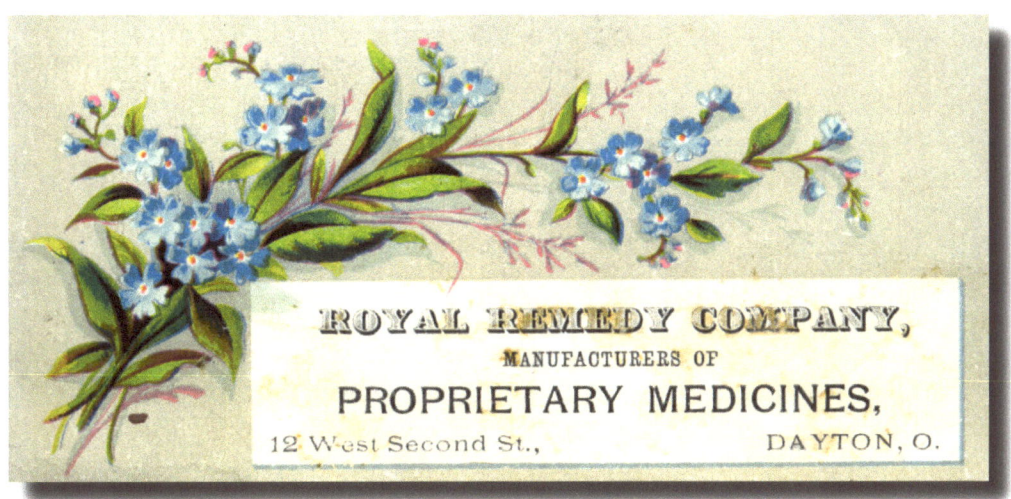

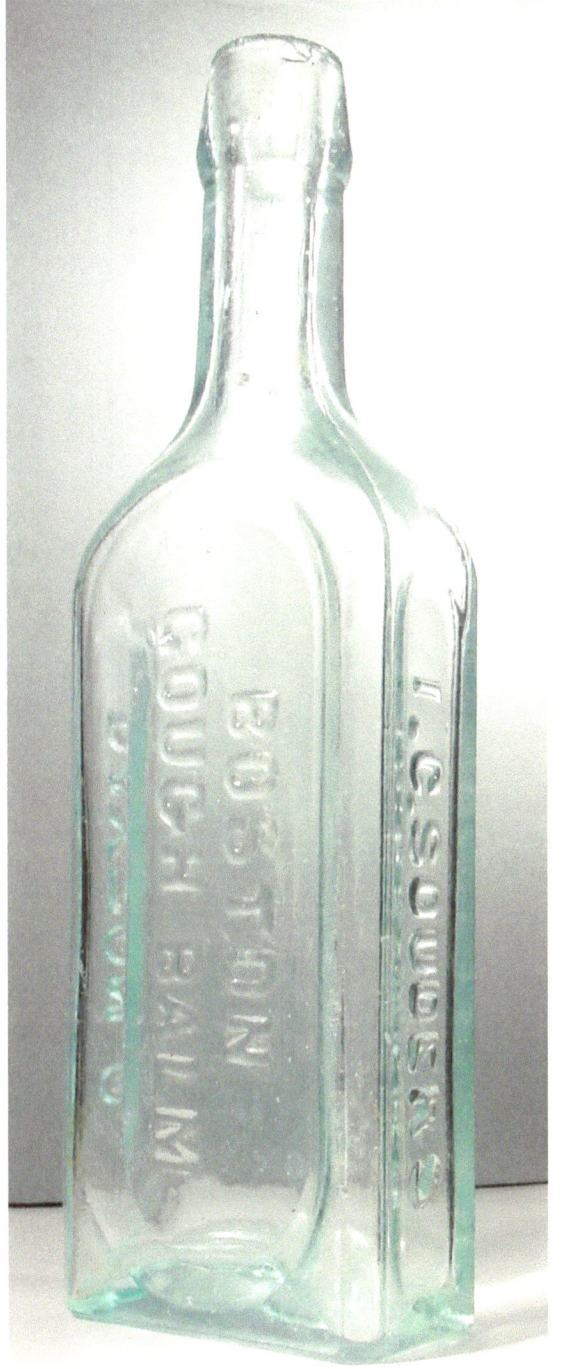

Boston Cough Balm

In 1876 Irvin C. Souders used his botanical knowledge as a nurseryman to create his "Boston Cough Balm", which he sold out of his home at 32 Blind Street. Souders claimed that his balm could cure both coughs and colds, as well as any type of throat infection. In 1880 Souders began selling under the name of the Royal Remedy Company and opened an office at 453 East 5th Street. Souders later hooked up with Hardman Anderson. Under this partnership the company expanded its product line to include flavoring extracts and perfumes. In 1888 the company incorporated under the name of Royal Remedy and Extract Company, moved into a three-story building at 21 East Second Street, and employed sixty workers to keep up with the demand for the new products.

As time passed, the medicinal line of products was eventually dropped. In 1905 Souders sold his interest in the company and opened a bakery. The Royal Remedy and Extract Company continued to sell flavoring extracts and chewing gum until 1931.

Potter's Plasters

The pitch about Potter's Plaster sort of went like this: In 1875 Ira A. Potter had been troubled with rheumatism for six years. Although he tried all kinds of medicines and different doctors, Potter continued to get worse. When he could not get out of bed alone, Potter decided to create a plaster (sort of a medicated bandage) with his own ingredients. After using this plaster for one week he found himself entirely cured. Potter made and gave the plasters away free until 1883, before placing them on the market. By this time he had experimented with different compounds to cure a variety of diseases, supposedly with great success. In 1890 he moved from New York to Dayton and began selling the plasters from his office at 8½ Brown Street. The plasters were advertised as being good for lame backs, rheumatism and even heart trouble. Potter continued to sell his plasters until his death in 1914.

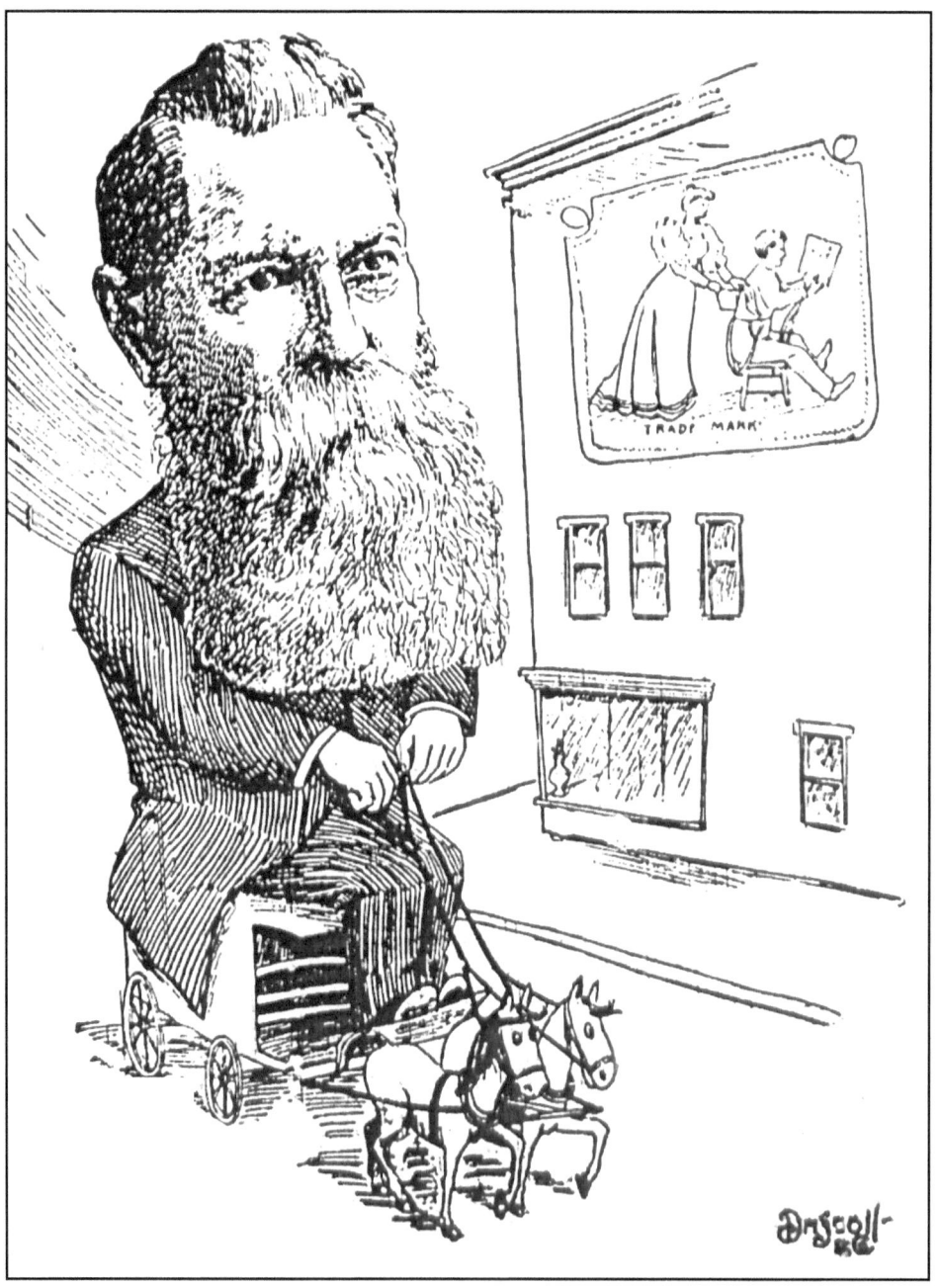

Ira A. Potter and his delivery wagon. Notice the company's trademark on the wall.

Ambition Tablets

Better known for his "Sarsaparilla" nostrum, Albert A. Hirsch's also manufactured "Ambition Tablets". Not only did the pills rid users of that tired feeling, giving "new life to Man and Woman", but was also supposedly effective for scrofula, piles, and rheumatism. As an added bonus it also cleared up unsightly pimples. Hirsch was in the nostrum business from 1895 to 1936.

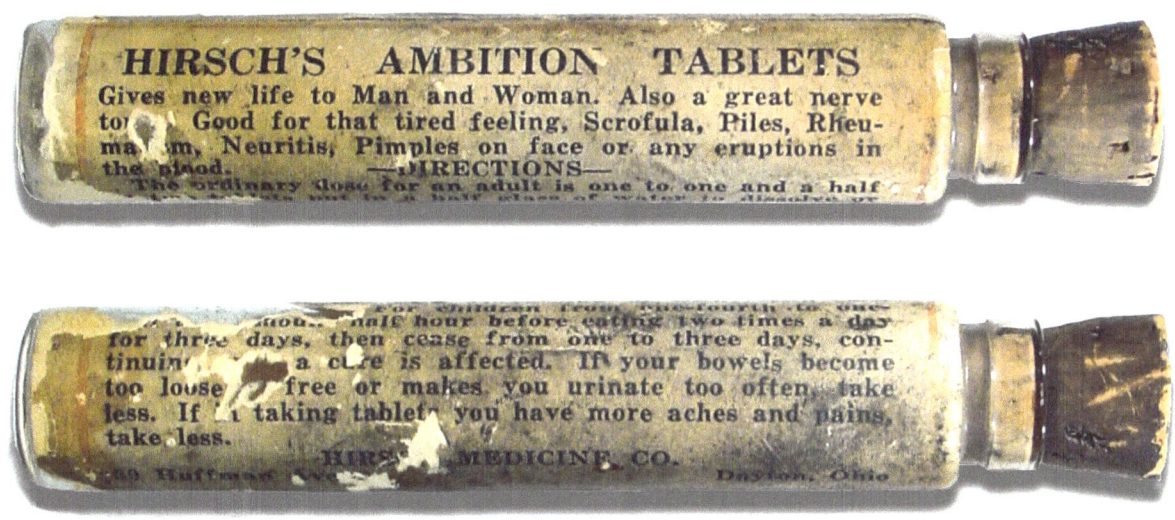

Dr. J. Kramer's Eye Salve

In 1880 S. N. Smith & Co., who had taken over Dr. Crook's business several years earlier, began offering "Dr. J. Kramer's German Eye Salve". Touted as a positive cure for weak and diseased eyes, the buyer was guaranteed that "no remedy is so immediate in its effects" to cure sore eyes. Buyers disagreed. Within a year the company quit producing Dr. Kramer's salve.

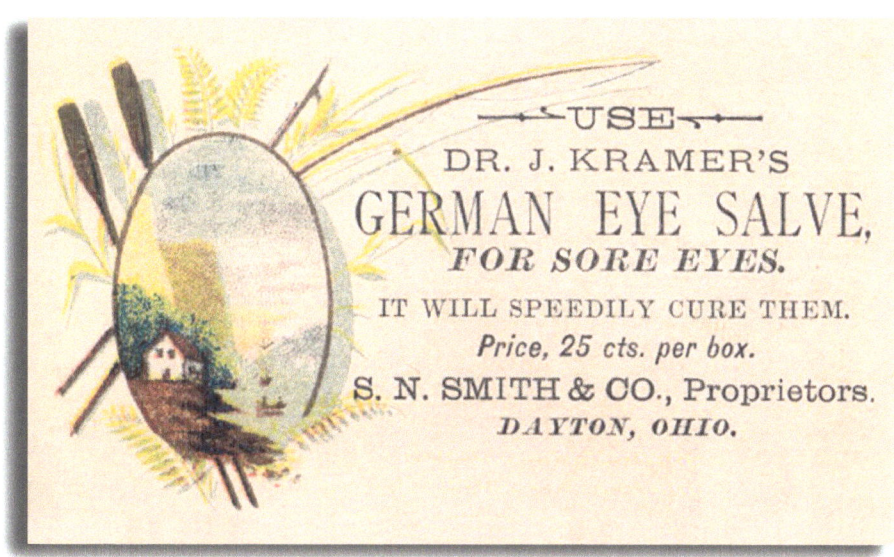

K-D Kidney Tablets

   The Redwood Medicine Company opened in 1926 in rooms at the rear of 1125 North Main Street. The company began offering K-D Tablets, a diuretic that gently stimulated the kidneys into removing "acid-forming, poison-generating products" from the blood and tissues. This enabled the users' system to overcome ailments such as pain in the back and loins, while also helping people who had a frequent desire to urinate. The following year The Redwood Medicine Company moved to the U.B. Building at the corner of 4th and Main Street, staying there until their doors closed in 1938.

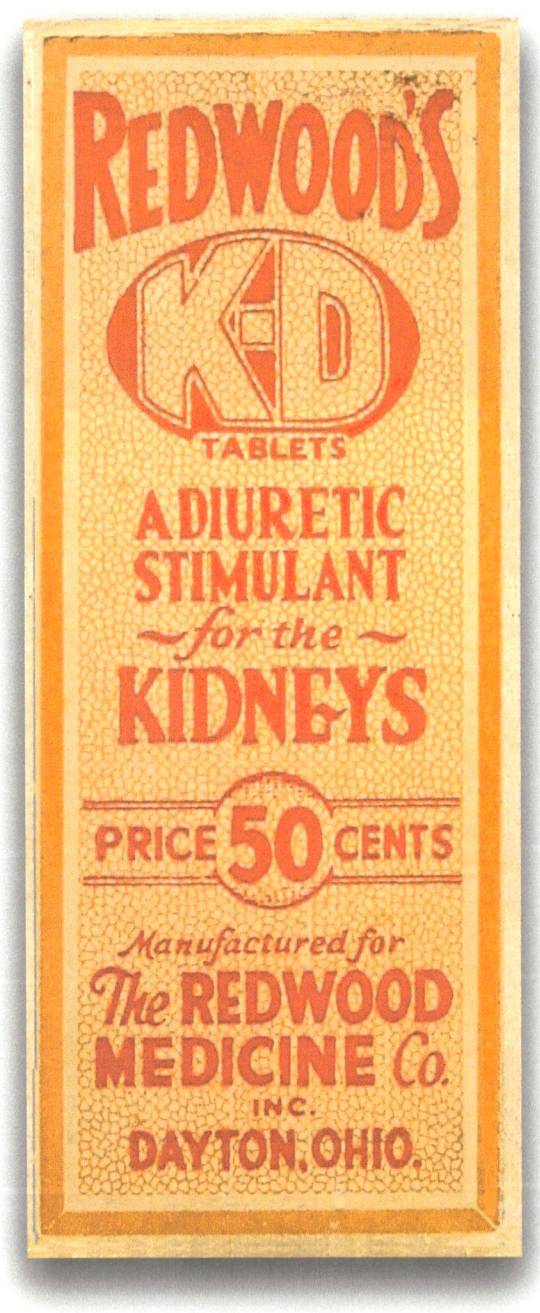
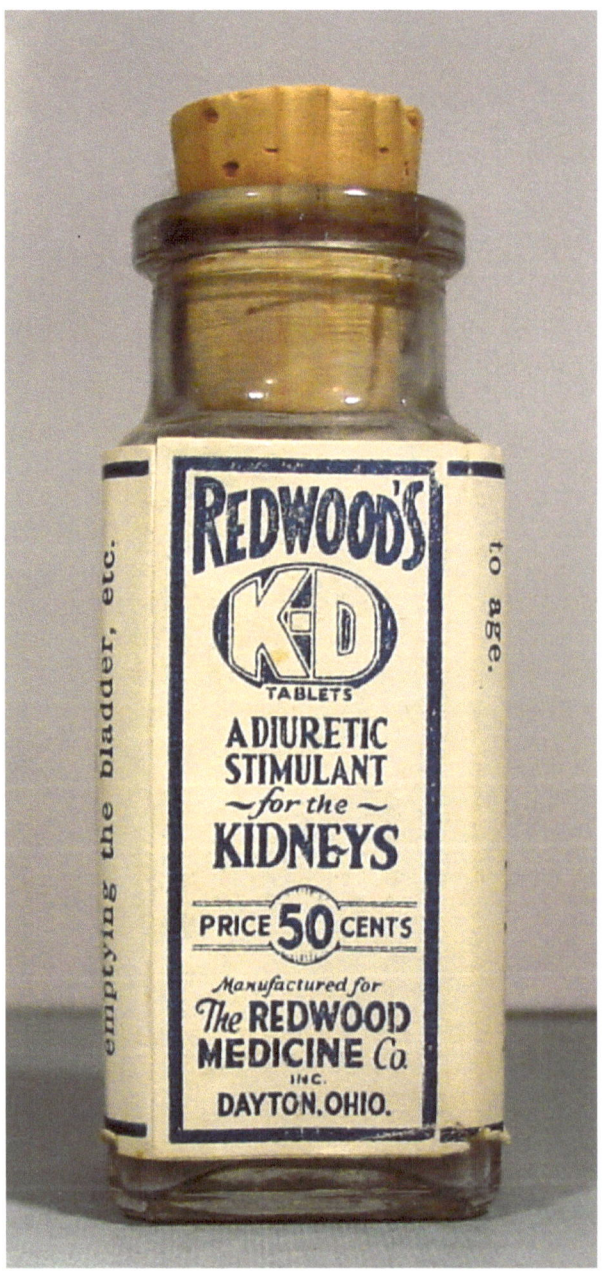

Redwood's Liniment

The Redwood Medicine Company also manufactured "Redwood's Liniment". Made of 95% alcohol, sufferers were directed to rub the liniment on any areas where they felt pain. It's likely that some buyers felt a pain in their throat and reached the affected area by drinking the remedy.

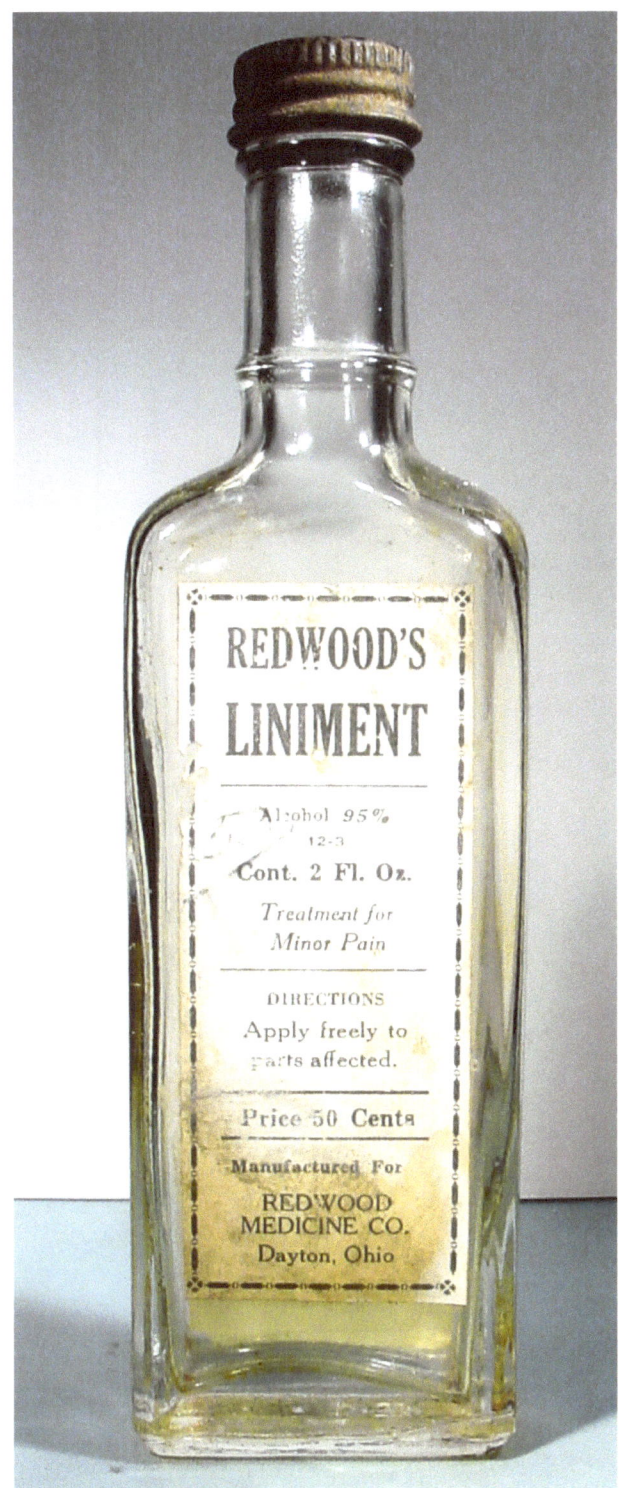

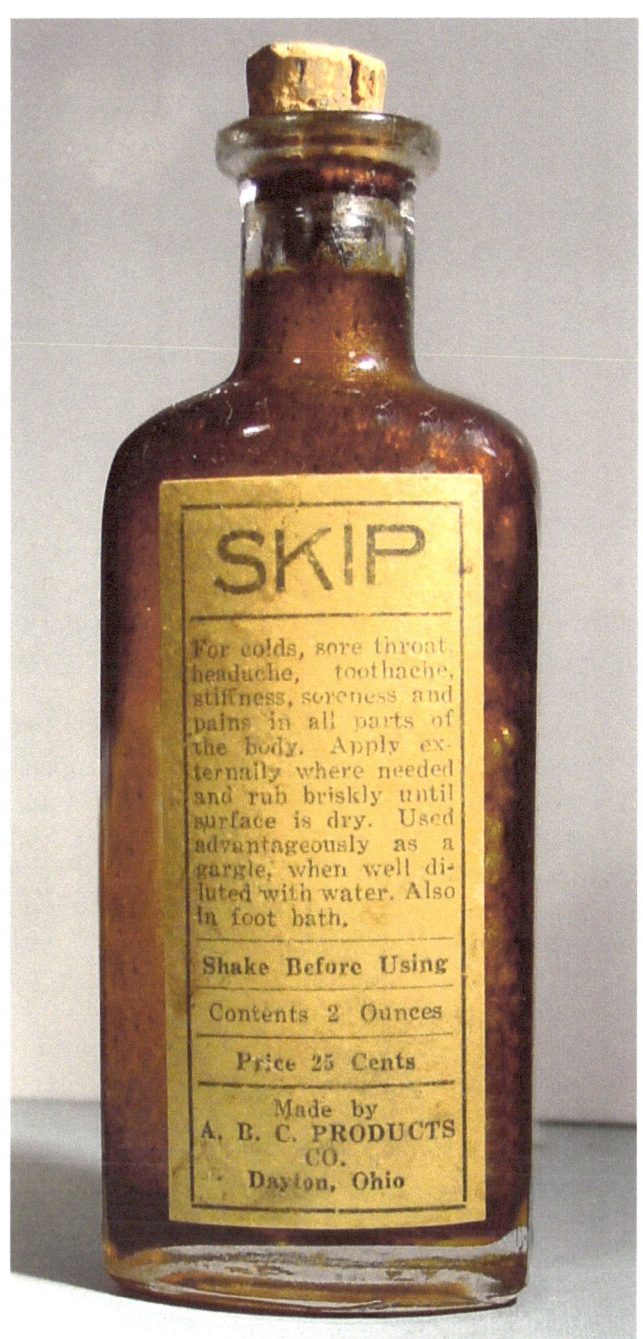

Skip

Not a lot is known about A.B.C. Products, but they did leave behind evidence of their existence in the form of the corked bottle that you see above. Their only known product was a nostrum called "SKIP". The brownish liquid concoction was to be rubbed briskly wherever needed, to help control the pains and sufferings of a sore throat, headache, toothache or all-around stiffness and soreness. It could also be mixed with water and used as a gargle or foot bath.

Low's Electric Liniment

Throughout the mid to late nineteenth century the public had a curiosity of electricity. There were electric salves, hairbrushes, ointments and even "electrified" food. It was thought that electricity could be used to draw out poisons like mercury out of the body. Others suggested that the gases from decaying food had a positive charge which caused a variety of diseases. It was thought that electricity could be used to create negative elements which would "consume" any undigested food in the body and allow a person to heal. The interest and misunderstanding of the mysterious aspects of electricity was encouraged by nostrum manufacturers.

In 1871 David B. Low took advantage of the fad and began manufacturing an "Electric Ointment" as a means of curing rheumatism, sprains, sore throat and other aches and pains of the body. The following year the company changed its name to Low Brothers, after Cornelius M. Low became a partner in the business. The company folded in 1875.

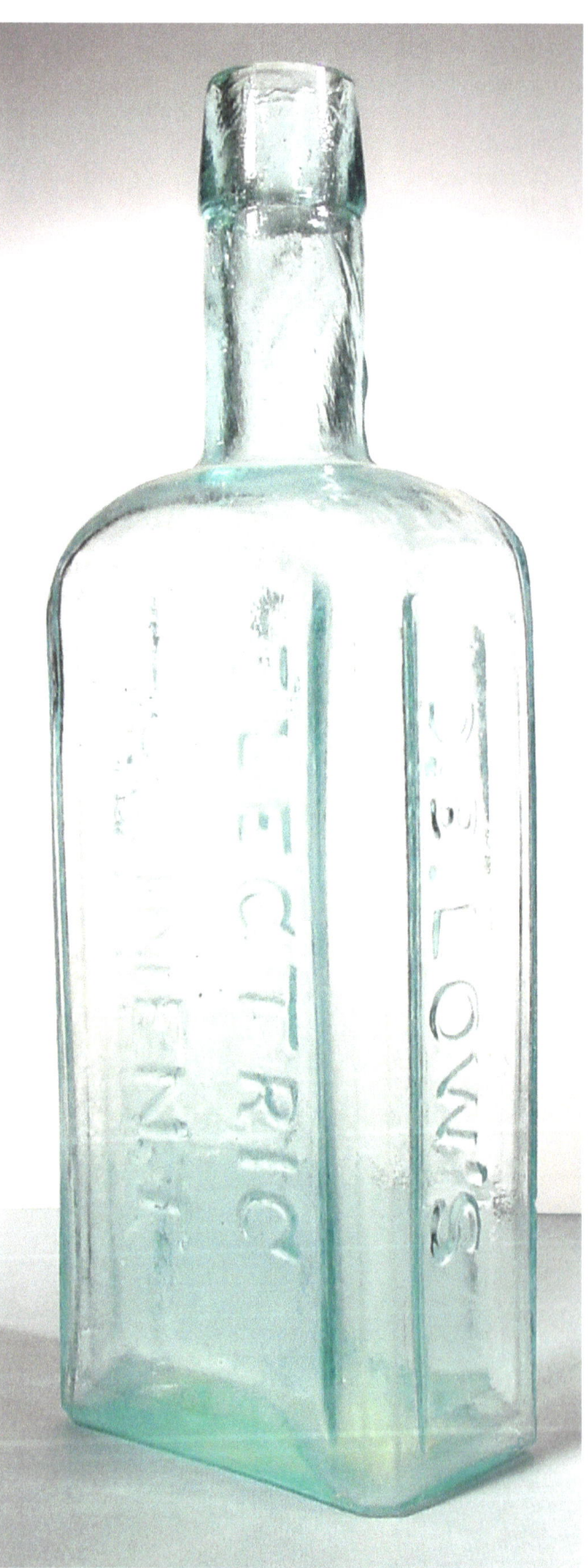

Continental Ointment

In 1909 the Continental Specialty Company was formed to manufacture and sell a salve they called "Continental Ointment". The salve's claim to fame was its ability to treat cuts, bites, bruises, burns, scalds, sunburn, eczema, sore throat, sore gums and other problems. Its motto was "The Marvelous Salve and Perfect Poultice for Horses and Humans". The same treatment that was used to obtain quick relief from an injury in humans "never fails to relieve animals from any skin or hoof trouble." Perhaps people didn't care to be compared with animals, or maybe the salve didn't work as well as buyers of it hoped. But for whatever reason, the company lasted only two years. The salve made a short comeback in 1916, with ads running in the Lancaster, Ohio newspaper. The company is not listed as having reopened during this period, so perhaps it was a last-ditch effort to get rid of remaining stock.

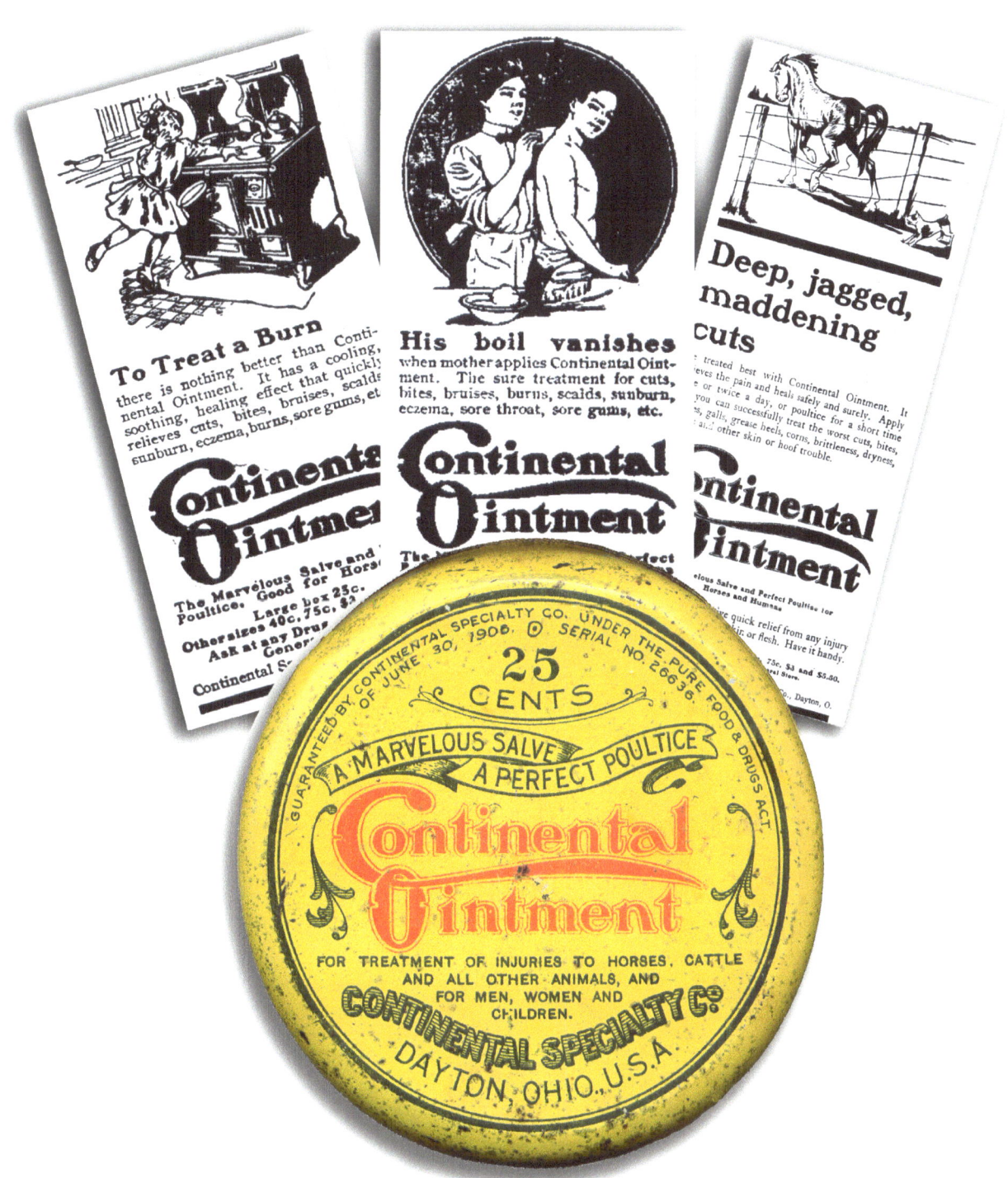

Chapter Eleven
Blackburn Products Company

The Blackburn Products Company first began as the Victory Remedy Company in rooms at the rear of 203 South Summit Street. Started by Ira Robert Blackburn in 1905, the company sold a preparation labeled "Blackburn's Castor-Oil-Pills", which was used to ease constipation. Soon after the Food and Drugs Act of 1906 was passed Blackburn was prosecuted by the government for shipping a misbranded drug product over the state line from Ohio to Michigan. According to an analysis made by the government labs, the pills contained barely a trace of castor oil, if any at all. As the cathartic, curative and therapeutic effects of castor oil were essentially "almost wholly absent", the use of the words castor oil was deemed unjustified and constituted misbranding. Blackburn pled guilty and paid the fine and costs of prosecution.

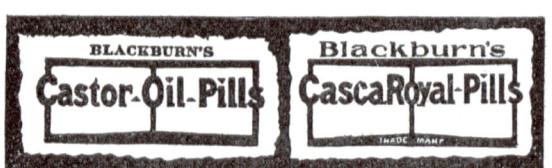

BEFORE AND AFTER
The Passage of the Food and Drugs Act.

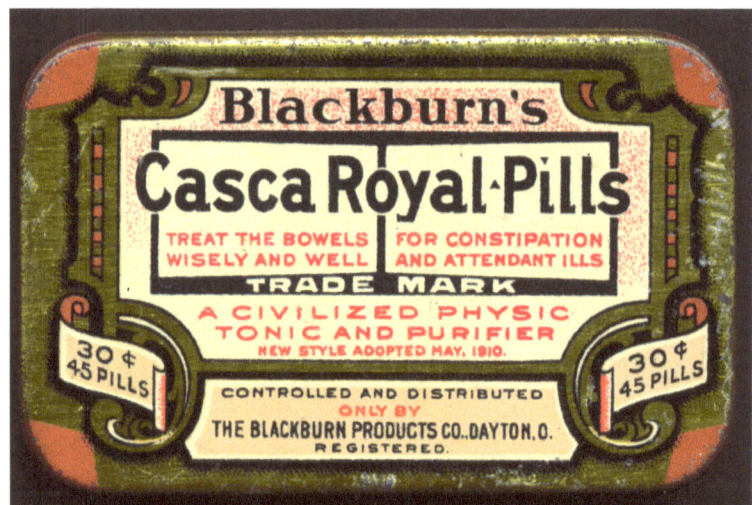

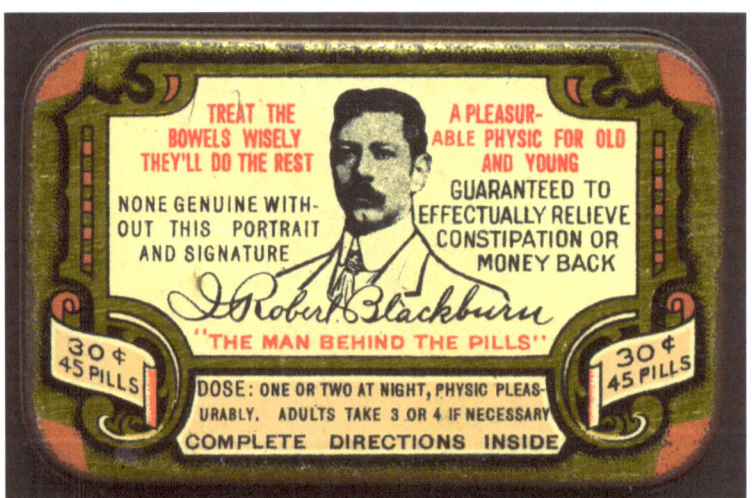

Starting in May 1910, I. Robert Blackburn's proud portrait adorned the back of every tin container of CascaRoyal-Pills.

The setback didn't stop Blackburn. On February 13, 1908 Blackburn Products Company was incorporated, with Ira Blackburn as president and John W. Miller as vice-president. The company moved to a new location on the northeast corner of 5th and Summit Street and began again. The castor oil pills were renamed "Blackburn's CascaRoyal-Pills." The business began introducing a number of health and beauty products, including nerve tonics, pain relievers and skin softeners. Within a year business had picked up to the point that the company moved to another new location, this time to 312 South College Street.

The Casca-Royal pills were merely the first of many products the company would offer the public over the next 40+ years.

Compound Fluid Balmwort

Compound Fluid Balmwort was recommended for those who suffered from a kidney disease. The liquid contained 16 per cent alcohol and the company recommended that 1 ounce of the Balmwort be mixed with 2 ounces of compound syrup of sarsaparilla and 2 ounces of gin. "Balmwort Tablets" were also sold by the company for the same health related issues, except that in advertising put out on the product, the company warned those afflicted with kidney disease to avoid alcohol! The public was urged to use Balmwort Tablets if urine was passed too frequently or not frequently enough, as well as when the urine had too much color and when it had too little. The company also stressed that anyone suffering from back pains could easily have diseased kidneys and not know it.

Vilane Powder

Vilane Powder was sold as a "concentrated powerful antiseptic germicide and disinfectant" and was recommended for treating hay fever, hemorrhages, tonsillitis and sore throats. After analyzing a sample of the powder, chemists in North Dakota reported that the mixture did not possess any germ-killing action at all. "As a germicide, this preparation is valueless and the claims made are absolutely false and misleading." Their findings were published in *The Journal of the American Medical Association,* April 13, 1912.

$1,000 Reward

UNDER OATH
If Blackburn's Casca Royal-Pills Contain Croton Oil in Any Form.

State of Ohio, County of Montgomery, ss.

To whom it may concern:—

Personally appeared before me, I, Robert Blackburn, who being duly sworn according to law deposes and says: That the proprietary remedy known to the public as Blackburn's Castor-Oil Pills, and lately as Blackburn's CascaRoyal-Pills, **do not now, and never did** contain one particle of Croton Oil in any form whatever; reports of incompetent (or grafter) chemists, to the contrary notwithstanding. He further says under oath that he will pay the sum of $1,000 to any doctor, chemist or private individual who can conclusively show by chemical and physiological tests that the pills above referred to do contain Croton Oil; or, that they do not contain Castor Oil.

I. Robert Blackburn.

Sworn to before me by the said I, Robert Blackburn and by himsubscribed in my presence this **8th day** of June, 1908.

JOSEPH A. WORTMAN,
Notary Public, Montgomery Co., Ohio.

NOTE:—I personally guarantee these pills to be a harmless, civilized, pleasurable physic and a true remedy for constipation.—I. R. B.

In 1908 Ira Robert Blackburn released this ad in numerous newspapers, from New York to Wisconsin, personally offering a $1000 reward to anyone who could prove that CascaRoyal-Pills did not contain castor oil. The ad also belittled any reports to the contrary, suggesting that the chemists who made those claims were either incompetent or being bought off.

Sulpherb Tablets

Sulpherb Tablets were touted as a laxative blood cleaner that aided digestion and relieved constipation. The tablets did indeed work well as a general laxative. This was sold under I. Robert Blackburn's other buiness, the Prescription Products Company, but it was eventually released as a nostrum of the Blackburn Product Company.

Mentho-Laxene Salve

Mentho-Laxene Salve was advertised as being triple the strength of regular salves on the market. It acted as an aid for congestion, sore throat and hay fever and could be used on inflamed muscles and joints. It also worked as a healing agent for burns, cuts and sores.

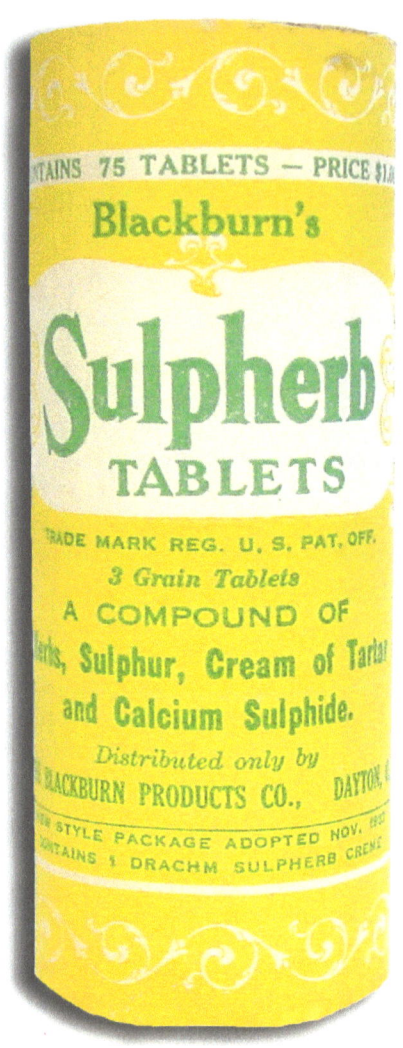

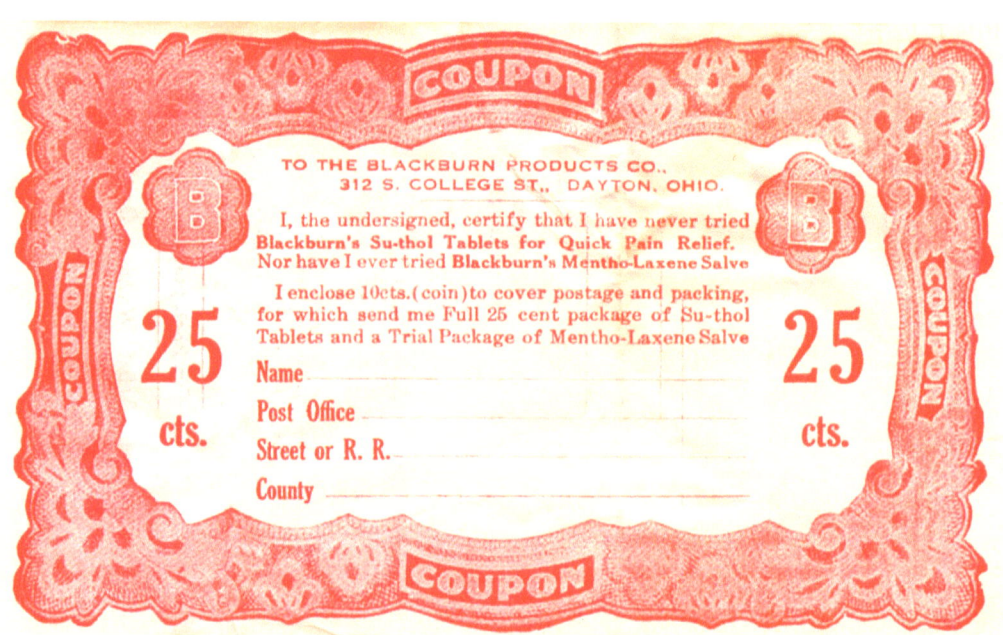

This 25 cent coupon was good for a free package of Su-Thol Tablets and a trial tube of Mentho-Laxene Salve. The coupon was placed in other Blackburn merchandise.

Essence of Mentho-Laxene

In 1916, I. Robert Blackburn found himself in court yet again. The focus this time was on one of the company's biggest sellers, a cough syrup known as "Essence of Mentho-Laxene." One pint of cough and cold medicine was made by mixing 2.5 ounces of Mentho-Laxene with one pint of granulated sugar and a half-pint of boiling water. The resulting mixture was also suppose to help relief sufferers of bronchitis and bronchial asthma and act as a preventative of consumption and la grippe. Federal chemists found that Mentho-Laxene was made up of 34 per cent alcohol together with ammonia salt, sugar and several other ingredients, none of which were effective for the claims being made. The company was found guilty of making false and fraudulent claims with reckless and wanton disregard of their truth or falsity. Blackburn Products was fined $50 and costs.

The company continued to prosper. Ira Robert Blackburn began using the profits to help Dayton's less fortunate. Described as an unassuming man who shunned personal publicity, Blackburn aided in the formation of the West Side Civic Association and the Dayton Advertising Club. Blackburn was also a hearty supporter of providing aid to the mentally ill. Along with Edward Davies, M. J. Gibbons and E. G. Burkam, Blackburn helped organize the Ohio Association for the Mentally Sick in 1931.

Ira Robert Blackburn retired from Blackburn Products Company in 1942 and the company moved its headquarters to 1652 Brown Street. On January 29, 1946 Blackburn passed away at the age of 72 and was buried at Woodland Cemetery. The Blackburn Products Company folded a year or two later.

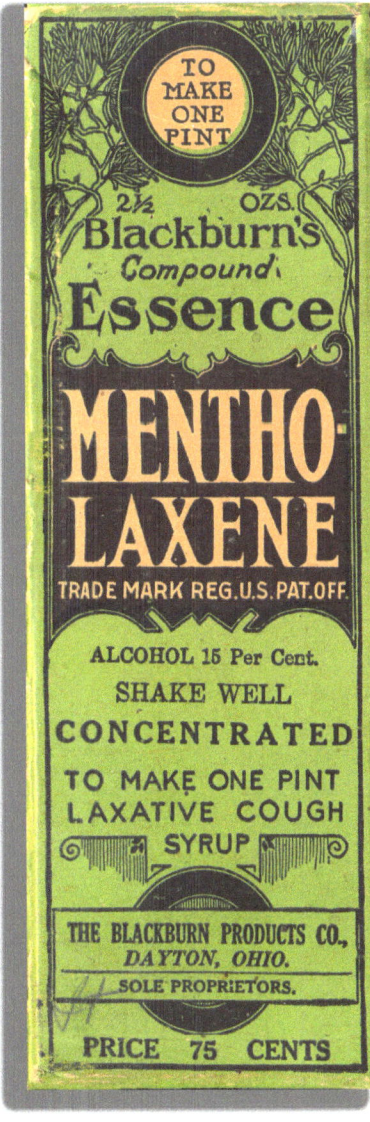
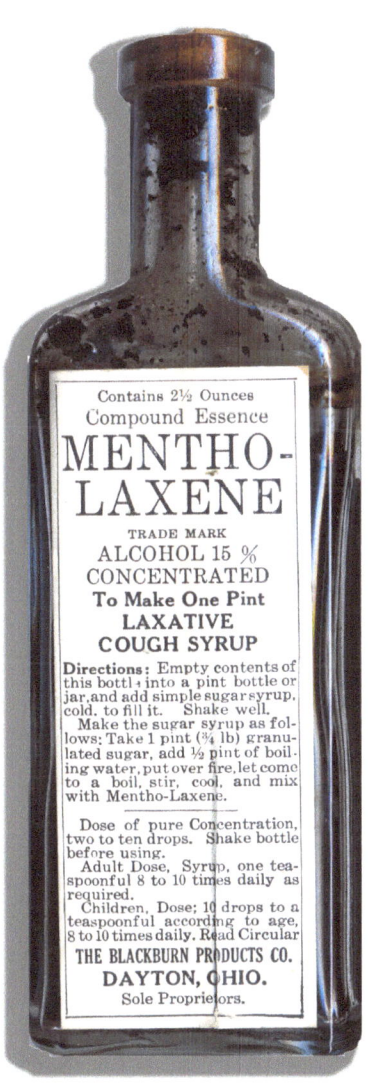

Selling Nostrums by the "Fake-Prescription Method"

One of the "features" of metropolitan newspapers at the turn of the century was a section called the "Health Department", in which would be given helpful hints on how readers should take care of themselves. Patent medicine manufacturers soon realized that these pages were a gold mine. They would run an ad that for all the world looked to be an advice column devoted to answering queries from readers regarding health issues. But the answers would often recommend a remedy that contained a nostrum, which would be referred to in a way that lead the unsuspecting reader to imagine that it was just another ordinary drug.

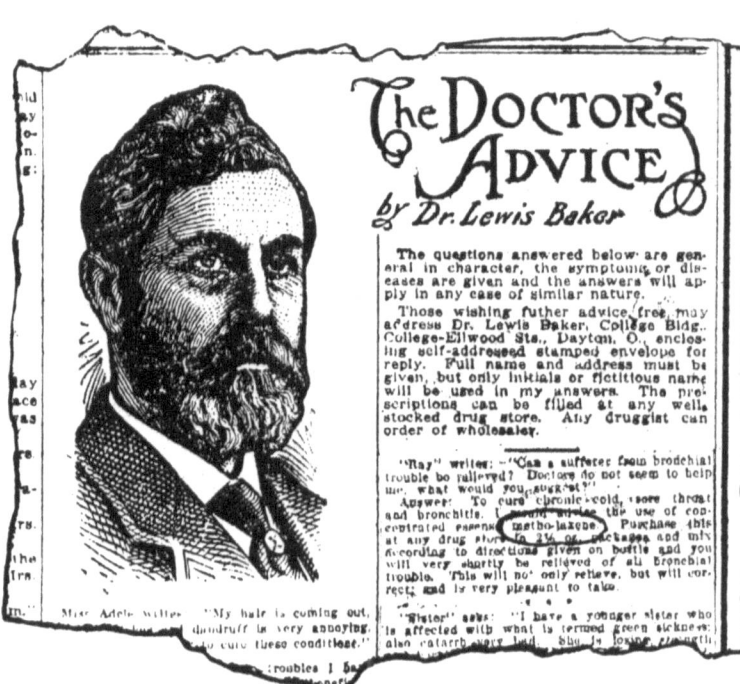

Blackburn Products Company sold a number of products by this "fake-prescription" method. Several newspapers across the country carried the column, entitled "The Doctor's Advice", in which Dr. Lewis Baker answers always recommended one or more of the patent medicines sold by the Blackburn Products Company, either alone or in combination with more legitimate drugs. For instance, this question and answer appeared in several newspapers on April 4, 1914.

P.P.C. writes: "If you can prescribe something to prevent an attack of appendicitis, please do so. I have constipation, sour stomach, headaches and am weak and listless with pains after eating."

Answer: "The best treatment for disordered stomach and bowels, due to indigestion, is tablets triopeptine, sold in sealed cartons with full instructions."

Triopeptine Tablets, of course, was a product sold by the Blackburn Products Company, a fact not mentioned in Dr. Baker's advice column. The tablets were sold to people who suffered from dyspepsia and indigestion. Each container held 60 tablets in three different colors. One or two red tablets were to be taken every morning immediately after breakfast, one or two white tablets after lunch and one or two blue tablets after the evening meal. Each type of color represented a different remedy and could be taken separately if needed. The red tablets helped reduce stomach acid, the white could be taken for belching and heartburn and the blue worked on intestinal pain and the passing of gas.

The column continued even after Dr. Baker's death in 1929. The masthead was changed to "Health Questions Answered" and the words "By the Late Dr. Lewis Baker's Associates" were added. Dr. Baker's bearded features would continue to be used until the column was dropped in the mid-1930s.

Health Questions Answered

By the Late Dr. Lewis Baker's Associates

An Advertisement

Telling How and When To Use Trustworthy Products and Reproducing Extracts of Patrons' Letters Relating to Cadomene, Balmwort, Sulpherb, Su-thol, Mentho-Laxene, Hypo-Nuclane, Triopeptine, Vilane, etc.

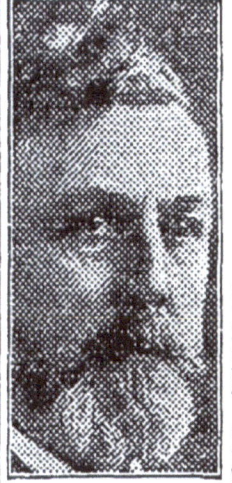

The Late Dr. Lewis Baker

TO THE LADIES: You will be overjoyed to know that there is now a remedy safe and dependable for the relief of the "muscular aches and pains" of the monthly period. This remedy, 5-grain Su-thol Tablets, is at once harmless, yet effective, and, of course, does not in any way obstruct the flow.

Taken at the approach of the period, and their use continued through it, these tablets provide escape from a single uncomfortable moment. If the pains have begun, they are relieved almost instantly.

Multitudes of women now use these tablets regularly each month, and, judging by their grateful letters and reports, they have proved a great contribution to women's welfare and comfort.

* * *

M. A. C. writes: "I feel tired all the time, have lost interest in my work and have a terribly depressed feeling. Have also lost weight and have become thin, pale and r..."

Answer: Suggest that Ca... Tablets be taken to aid improv... of both quality and quantity o... blood, thus restoring the n... functioning of the body organs... nervous system.

* * *

Mrs. G. G. writes: "We are a famil... of six. Recently, we all suffered with an epidemic of colds, which left all but Joseph, our oldest boy, with stubborn coughs. Have tried three different cough medicines, but relief has been only temporary."

Answer: To quickly relieve coughs due to colds, obtain Essence Mentho-Laxene, and use as per directions. As for the colds, try treating them with Mentho-Laxene Salve. You will find it affords remarkably prompt relief.

exceptionally effective in relieving and overcoming such symptoms.

A. T. O. writes: "Have used one particular laxative for several years, but it is now losing its effectiveness. Can you suggest a good one? One that don't gripe."

Answer: Believe you will find Casca-Royal Pills an ideal laxative, particularly superior in their gentleness.

* * *

O. C. C. writes: "Just plain indigestion is my trouble, with belching, bloating and formation of much gas after eating. Have tried two dyspepsia remedies without much relief."

Answer: Procure Triopeptine Tablets and take as per directions. Also regulate diet by finding out what does and does not agree with you.

* * *

Answer to Mrs. A. C. F.: For limbering up stiff, sore, swollen joints, nothing quite equals Mentho-Laxene Salve. Try it.

* * *

W. H. asks: "Have catarrh... nose and upper sinus... constantly dropping... giving me a ch... will help...

ing two boxes, my face began to clear up and by the time I had taken four boxes, my face was completely healed. That was four years ago. About a month ago, my face began breaking out again and this time before finishing one box, the pimples disappeared. So you can see why I say Sulpherb tablets are worth their weight in gold to me." (Signed) Flora Richardson, Box 68.

* * *

Mr. Burns Praises Balmwort

NEW YORK CITY, Martin Burns, 422 East 138 St., writes: "I have been using your Balmwort tablets for some time for urinary trouble, and it has helped me wonderfully. Before using, I had to get up 4 and 5 times at night and then had considerable trouble voiding. My family is using your Mentho-Laxene cough medicine and it is helping them the best of anything ever used, etc."

* * *

Mentho-Laxene Best for Coughs

NORTH EASTON, MASS., Mrs. W. P. Holbrook, 3 Howland Court, writes: "For a number of years we have used your Mentho-Laxene cough syrup, and we find it superior to any other we have had. The S... Tablets are all you claim f... present. We find Casca-... They quiet the nerves where ...nd your other remedies in ... store and we never fail to ...m to our friends."

...iracle for Indigestion

...PA., Joseph McKinley, ...: "I feel so happy to ...that I cannot rest ...few lines, thanking ...e' Triopeptine Tab-...because after suffer-...r five years and ...ey I earned with ...purchased Trio-...ho tablets as di-...egan to feel like ...packages. The ...y pocket for 3 ...them, but to ...s indigestion ...d in weight

A copy of Dr. Baker's "Health and Beauty" guide book could be had for a dollar. Advertised as containing helpful information on such topics as health and beauty secrets, love, courtship and marriage, it was mostly 128 pages of advice on how products from the Blackburn Products Company could help with all of life's little problems.

Health and Beauty

By LEWIS BAKER, M.D.
And Associate

An Explanation of Some of the Ailments that Affect Mankind

With Suggestions for Treatment of Simple or Minor Cases

Price $1.00

Chapter Twelve
Unmentionable Ailments

Many of the patent medicines offered at the turn of the century dealt with sexual disorders. The overwhelming majority of these were directed to women as remedies for "female complaints" a term which at first referred to menstrual irregularities, but which soon became a euphemism for abortion.

Henry Sewill, a member of the British Medical Association, wrote of how women had more of a tendency to trust those who promised to help them with their "difficulties."

> *Among the victims to quackery of every sort, women far outnumber men. They are always more trustful and, as a rule find it more difficult, especially when suffering, to believe that anyone can be base enough to abuse their confidence, mush less to take advantage of their helplessness in order to plunder and injure them.*

Much of the success of the "female regulator" medicines was also due to women not wanting to go to a male doctor, especially for certain problems, for obvious reasons. Women turned to other women, if they could, or to ordering the medication by mail.

F. Beard's Female Regulator

The F. Beard Company offered women with irregular periods a pill called "Superb". The company seems to have started in Louisville, Kentucky in 1903. By 1909 the company had moved to Dayton and had begun placing ads in the classified columns of nearby newspapers to drum up business. A typical ad would ask for ladies to send 25 cents for a catalog called "Secrets for Women" and a box of "Dr. Baird's Remedy". Those who sent a quarter received a batch of advertising of the various remedies of the F. Beard Company and a small wooden box containing some black pills. One of the circulars urged women to "send immediately for Superb Pills No. 3" if the sample in the box "does not bring about the monthly flow." According to the leaflet, Superb No. 3, now triple the strength of the original pill, was "made expressly for long-standing and aggravated cases" of women who had trouble maintaining their "monthly regularity." The company guaranteed that, if taken each month, the pill would prevent these irregularities and save the woman both worry and pain. The price of five dollars a box was asked.

> **LADIES**—Send 25c; Catalogue Secrets for Women and Box Dr. Baird's Remedy. Safe, Speedy, Regular. F. Beard Co., Dayton, O.

The company was actually owned by a man by the name of Oliver P. Beard who named the business after his wife, Frances. Although charging $5 for what should have been a $1 cure was almost on the order of extortion, many of the women had no one else to turn to. Mr. Beard knew his customers would gladly pay extra for the advice of another woman and the option of receiving a cure for their problem without having to talk to anyone face to face.

On October 4, 1913, *The Journal of the American Medical Association* warned its readers of the scam. Word must have gotten around quickly, for shortly thereafter the company was out of business.

Dr. DuChoine's Female Regulating Pills

The Dr. Harter Medicine Company offered "Dr. DuChoine's Female Regulating Pills". Developed for those troubled by irregular periods, the pills were "strengthening to the entire system (and) imparts tone, vigor and magnetic force to all functions of body and mind." From one to three tablets were to be taken three times a day, one hour before meals. The treatment was to begin two to three days before the period was to begin and continued until the "desired flow" was established.

In 1893 instructions for the pills included a warning for pregnant women not to use the medication during any period of pregnancy, as it could cause a miscarriage. Then the company added, in italic type *"We mean just what we say by this Caution, and no more."* It seems the company wanted to make it clear that it was only cautioning the use of its product, not advising that it should be used as an abortion pill.

WOMANLY BEAUTY

Is frequently destroyed by Female Complaints. Their efforts to appear pleasing and beautiful will prove of no avail when such conditions exist. Woman's beauty depends largely on good health, and cannot exist when she is afflicted with female irregularities, which are a protest against nature and deprive her of sexual rights, privileges and enjoyments, and completely unfit her for the companionship of man. Unfortunate indeed are the women who are troubled with Whites, Gleet, Seminal Weakness, Impotency or Barrenness, and all kindred ailments arising from a disordered state of the genital organs. Whatever may be the cause they will find in **Dr. Du Choine's Female Pills** a remedy that has no equal for the relief and cure of all diseases peculiar to their sex. We advise

Every Woman Who is Weak,

nervous and discouraged, particularly those who have thin, pale lips, cold hands and feet, and who are without strength and ambition, to use **Dr. Harter's Iron Tonic** in connection with **Dr. Du Choine's Female Regulating Pills**. These two incomparable remedies are women's best friend because they give strength to the body, induce refreshing sleep, improve the quality of the blood, quiet the nerves, purify the blood and brighten the complexion. They will cure the worst form of female complaints, falling and displacement, and consequent weakness, and are particularly adapted for the change of life. They will positively regulate the monthly periods and cause them to pass without pain.

The Change in Female Life

from girlhood to womanhood either results in health and happiness or disease and misery. How important it is, then, that mothers should look to the welfare of their daughters and see that they are properly instructed and protected during this critical period. Regular monthly uterine action is necessary to every woman's health. Ladies who are familiar with the benefits derived from the use of **Dr. Du Choine's Female Regulating Pills** recognize them as the only sure guide to menstrual regularity. This knowledge and confidence, gained by actual trial and use, accounts for their ability to constantly appear in public, at balls, parties, the opera, and entertainments of various kinds at which the

Women of Fashion

are expected to be present. Female irregularities are varied and may be constitutional, or the result of carelessness and neglect. They may follow a cold, and are often of the most positive and decided character, and unless met with a remedy that is safe and certain to cure, usually terminate fatally.

The monthly secretion must continue from maturity to the turn of life without unnatural obstructions. This is a demand of nature that must not be violated. Many ladies suffer at each monthly period, others at the commencement of menstruation. Occasionally the menstrual flow is too little, sometimes too much and attended with pain. Again it may be checked or changed in appearance; at first gradually and scarcely noticeable, yet the sufferer will be

The Victim

of ailments with which she has not been accustomed, and which will cause her much trouble, and perhaps a spell of sickness if not promptly relieved. Pregnant women should not use these pills during any period of pregnancy as they might produce a miscarriage, which is always attended with more or less danger. Sometimes a very slight cause will bring them on, hence the necessity of caution in the use of any medicine under such circumstances.

Dr. Du Choine's Female Regulating Pills are put up in small plain packages, securely sealed and sent by mail to any address on receipt of price, $1.00, or six bottles for $5.00; in currency, stamps, express or Post Office Orders.

Beware of Imitations as there are Many on the Market.

Moberly, Mo., July 15, 1894.
Gentlemen:—I have taken your **Dr. Du Choine's Female Regulating Pills** with the greatest satisfaction. Respectfully,
Mrs. Clara Walker.

Urbana, Ill., Feb. 10, 1895.
Gentlemen:—I have tried your **Dr. Du Choine's Female Regulating Pills** and find them excellent. Yours very truly,
Mrs. C. H. Maxwell.

Cedarville, Va., Feb. 4, 1895.
Dear Sirs:—A year ago I took two bottles of your **Dr. Du Choine's Female Regulating Pills**, and they did me more good than any other medicine I ever used. Very truly,
Mrs. A. Johnson.

Cottonwood Falls, Kan., June 17, 1894.
Gentlemen:—My wife desires a bottle of **Dr. Du Choine's Female Regulating Pills**, for which I enclose the money. She is a nurse, and has had excellent success with them. She has nothing but words of the highest praise for them. Yours very truly,
Henry Johnson.

Way Cross, Ga., Feb. 16, 1894.
Gentlemen:—Please send me a bottle of **Dr. Du Choine's Female Regulating Pills**, for which you will find money enclosed. I have taken one bottle and am wonderfully relieved. Very truly yours,
Tyva Barnard.

1897 ad for Dr. DuChoine's Female Regulating Pills.

Su-Thol Tablets

The Blackburn Products Company sold several products especially made for women. Su-Thol Tablets, (pronounced sooth-all), guaranteed quick relief from pain without the use of harmful narcotics such as cocaine, cannabis, opium or morphine. Although promoted for use with headaches, toothaches and backaches, it was also formulated to help with the "pain and suffering that comes to womanhood at certain times." Spending just a quarter for a package of fifteen tablets could relieve these "periodic pains of womanhood".

Mrs. J. E. Sweetman, of 1400 Huffman Avenue in Dayton, wrote the company to say how grateful she was.

For years I have had to go to bed each month on account of dreadful sickening pain. I had tried many pain remedies and would get some relief - but weakness followed for several days and my stomach rebelled. Your Suthol Tablets have stopped all pains. I do not have to go to bed, and now I scarcely notice the occasion. I just take a Suthol a day or two before and do not suffer at all. They do not weaken me or sicken me like other pain tablets did.

Cadomene Tablets

The Blackburn Products Company also manufactured Cadomene Tablets, for women who suffered from anemia. Symptoms of this condition included a loss of appetite, feeling "run down" or weak and the inability to get a good night's sleep. If past 40, the company warned that the troubles could also be the beginning of the "Change of Life." Left untreated, the condition could lead to hysteria, severe headaches, rheumatism, gloomy thoughts and even a "Nervous Breakdown." Fortunately, each Cadomene tablet contained phosphates, iron, phosphorus and sulphates, "elements essential to rebuild the anemic blood...tone up the digestive organs and allay the nerve irritation." In case the point was missed, ads would show a picture of a man looking into the eyes of his wife, with the lines:

The tired feeling has vanished, and in its place is energy... Work becomes pleasure, pleasure becomes joy and joy becomes ecstasy.

Another, very important warning was given to mothers whose daughters were entering womanhood. It was claimed that many young girls became "broken down in health" at this time of their lives, a tragedy that could mar their future health and happiness. The real danger came from a condition called chlorosis, sometimes known as the "Green Sickness." Irregular and excessive monthly periods could cause a drain on the system, leaving sufferers with a pale, greenish complexion, severe headaches, nausea and indigestion. It was suggested that mothers give their daughters Cadomene tablets for several weeks in order to help them produce "plenty of rich red blood" and build up the weakened system.

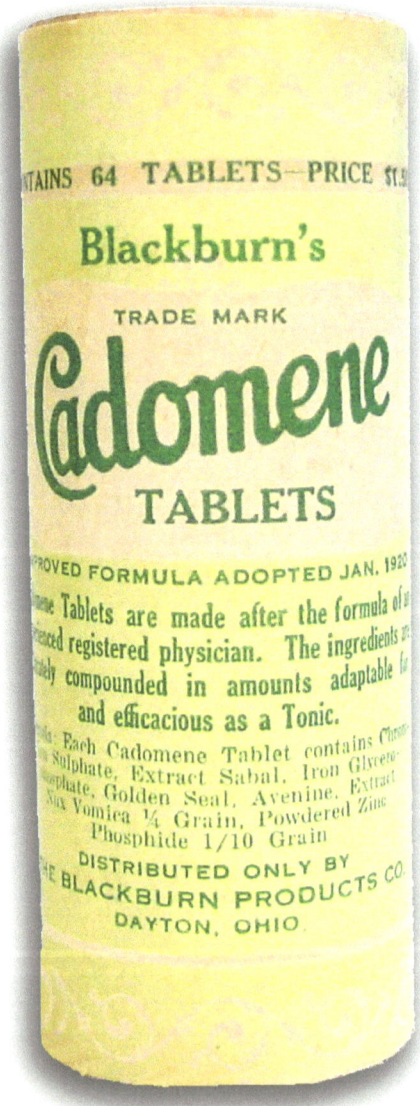

Men had a sexual problem of their own that they were too embarrassed to talk about, the fear of disease or insanity from masturbating. In 1892, the Dictionary of Psychological Medicine described the effects of masturbation as "moral and mental shipwreck, the whole nature is deteriorated.... mental faculties become blunted.... The miserable wretch would commit suicide if he dared, but rarely has the courage . . . and sinks into melancholic dementia."

In 1911 Ivan Bloch, author of *Sexual Life in England*, wrote that "In the treatment of masturbation, the methods of the older physicians who appeared before the child armed with great knives and scissors and threatened a painful operation or even to cut off the genital organs may often be used and often effect a radical cure."

Fortunately, there were less drastic solutions.

Dr. DuChoine's Nerve Pills

The Dr. Harter Medicine Company's ad for their "Dr. DuChoine's Nerve Pills" was quite blunt in who needed their product, and why.

To Young Men... Did it ever occur to you that your vices were known to the world? The intelligent person reads in the expression of your face the truths you in vain attempt to hide. Nature abused asserts her rights and makes plain to the world your most secret vices. You alone are to blame for your unfortunate condition and for not seeking a remedy that will restore your health and manhood. Dr. DuChoine's Nerve Pills is the best known remedy for the speedy relief and cure of sexual weakness and physical disability. They may confidently be relied upon by those who have a remnant of manhood remaining.

Symptoms that a person had the "disease" included a loss of appetite, lack of energy, weak eyes, over-sensitivity of the "sexual system" and pimples; characteristics linked at the time to the curse of masturbation.

At $2 a bottle, the pills were double that charged by other companies for the same type of medication. However, the company claimed that the price wasn't exorbitant at all.

The materials (of the pills) are expensive, and they are prepared in the most scientific manner. Considering the nature of the medicine, what the patient has at stake, and comparing price with the price of treatment charged by doctors who make a specialty of such diseases, Dr. DuChoine's Pills are exceedingly low priced.

The company guaranteed that the neighbors wouldn't know what had been sent for, the pills being sent in a securely sealed, plainly wrapped package.

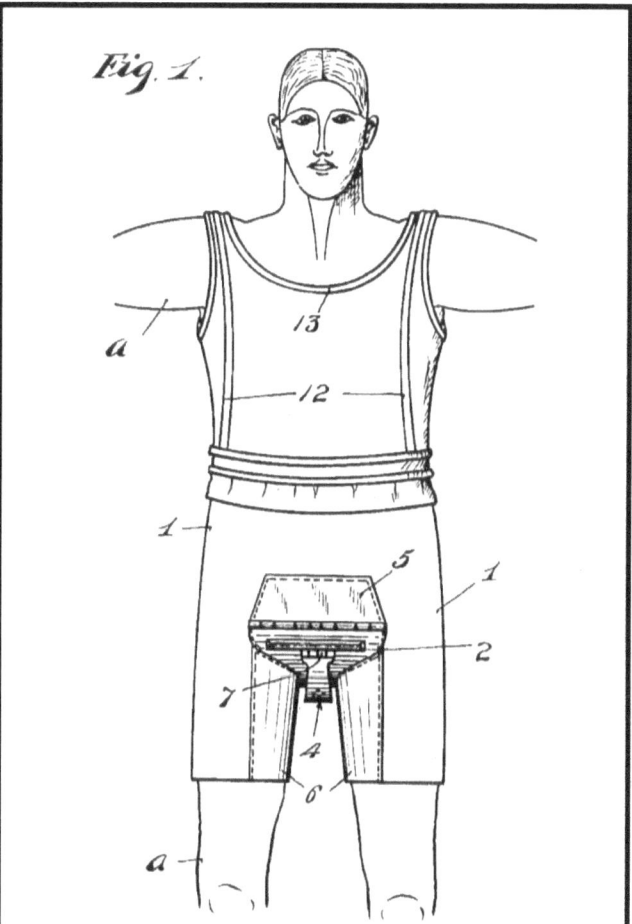

From 1856 to 1932 the U.S. Patent Office awarded 33 patents for devices that prevented masturbation. Ellen E. Perkins, a nurse from Beaver Bay, Minnesota, applied for a patent on a device she called "Sexual Armor". She stated that the garment was important due to the "deplorable but well known fact that one of the most common causes of insanity, imbecility and feeble mindedness, especially in youth, is due to masturbation, or self abuse." The imbeciles at the Patent Office must have agreed, for she was awarded Patent #875,845 in 1908.

Vegetable Syphilitic Remedy

Syphilis was once known as the "great imitator" due to its mimicking other diseases. Symptoms included stomach cramps, headaches, depression and heart problems. If left unchecked, the disease could cause the bridge of the nose to collapse, leaving a very deformed hole in the center of the face.

With so many symptoms, it was natural for most men who had dallied in their youth to believe that every headache or stomach pain was a sure sign that they had syphilis. Patent medicine sellers played on this fear, offering cures for a condition that at the time was uncurable.

Dr. Oliver Crook's remedy for the dreaded disease was advertised in the newspapers as "Vegetable S-PH-L-S Remedy." Potential customers could write for a description of the disease and the disorders it caused. If they found that they needed the cure, it could be obtained for the high price of $3 a bottle.

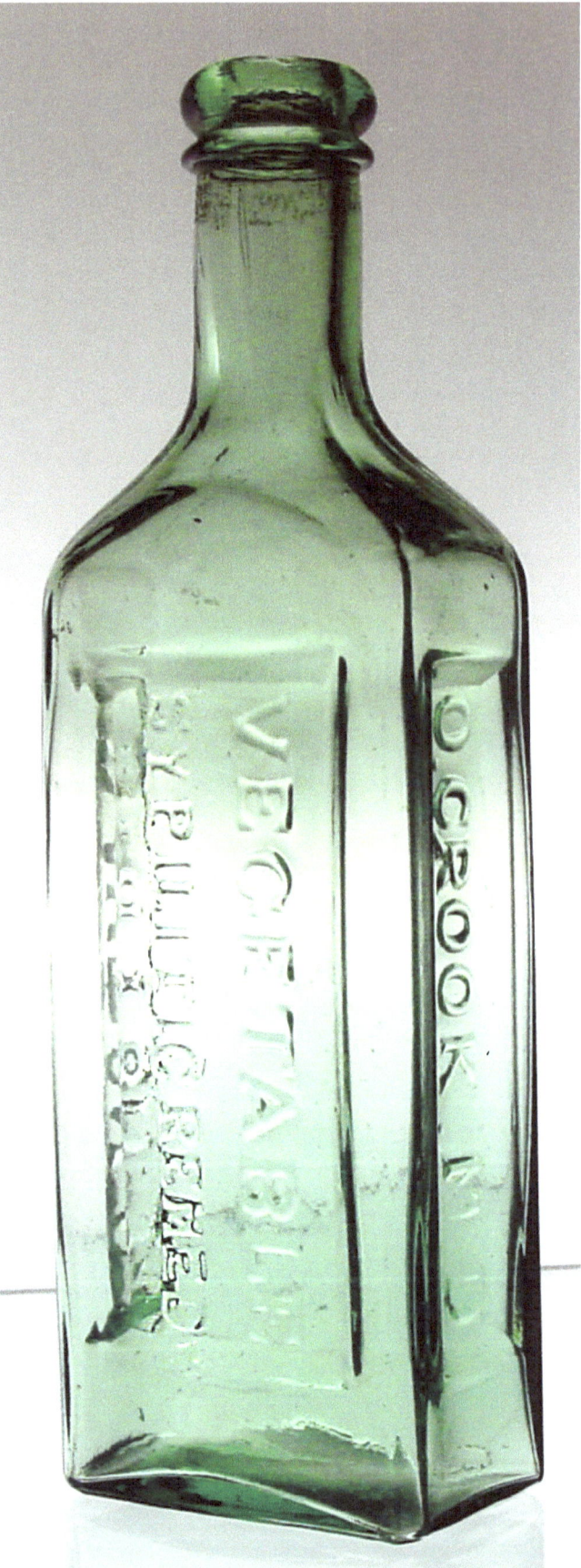

S.yPH.L.S

DR. CROOK'S
VEGETABLE
S-PH-L-S REMEDY,
Will positively cure
SYPHILIS It any stage,
Or any Disease entailed by it.

It will become the Standard Remedy.

There never was such a remedy to eradicate every particle of Syphilitic poison. It has never been known to fail; requires no change of diet; is agreeable to the taste; cures speedily and effectually, and cannot injure.

Physicians learned and skillful in the treatment of other diseases have sought in vain for a specific for Syphilis (Pox), and utterly failed in its treatment.

Hence we place our medicine within the reach of the afflicted to save them by its healing power from a life of suffering and sorrow.

Send for a Pamphlet.

Dr Crook's S-ph-l-s Remedy is sold by all Druggists, $3.00 per bottle.

Full directions accompany every bottle.

DR. OLIVER CROOK & CO.,
690-1y   Proprietors.

Chapter Thirteen
Vanity Nostrums

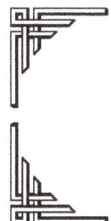
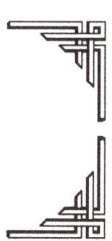

Although the curse of having poor skin, being too fat, losing ones hair or being flat chested is not a disease, the patent medicine companies were quite able to convince people otherwise.

The Blackburn Products Company was the most popular producer and seller of vanity cures in Dayton. The Prescription Products Company and the Leslie Company were two other businesses connected with Ira Robert Blackburn used to market these types of products. Just like Blackburn's medical line, their vanity remedies were chiefly advertised under what was called the "fake-prescription" method, in this instance in an advice column written by Claire Ainsworth. The column was usually placed in the "Answers to Correspondents" section of the newspaper under the title "How to be Beautiful - Secrets of Health and Beauty." Each "answer" recommended one or more of nostrums sold by the Blackburn Products Company, Prescription Products Company or Leslie Company.

Skin Products

Clogged pores didn't cause pimples, "bad blood" or ulcers did. Claire Ainsworth recommended several types of treatments, depending on the condition of the skin. "Quinoxide Tablets" worked as a blood purifier, rid the face of pimples and whitened the skin. Massaged into the skin, "Gloriol Tonique Astringent" helped firm flabby cheeks, double chins and ugly wrinkles. "Hypo-Nuclane" was endorsed as a way to improve the blood and give color to the complexion. "Rose-Kayloin" was a preparation for use as both a pimple and freckle remover. The thought was that people afflicted with chronic ulcers and constipation would sometimes absorb the poisons of fermented food into their blood. This would manifest itself in the form of pimples, skin ulcers and itchy skin. Readers were told to mix Rose-Kayloin with lanolin, then place the ointment on the skin to help heal sores.

According to a report made in 1915 by the Connecticut Agricultural Experiment Station, Rose-Kayloin was essentially sulphur and potassium carbonate with small amounts of sodium carbonate and sulphur compounds, more or less the ingredients found in soap.

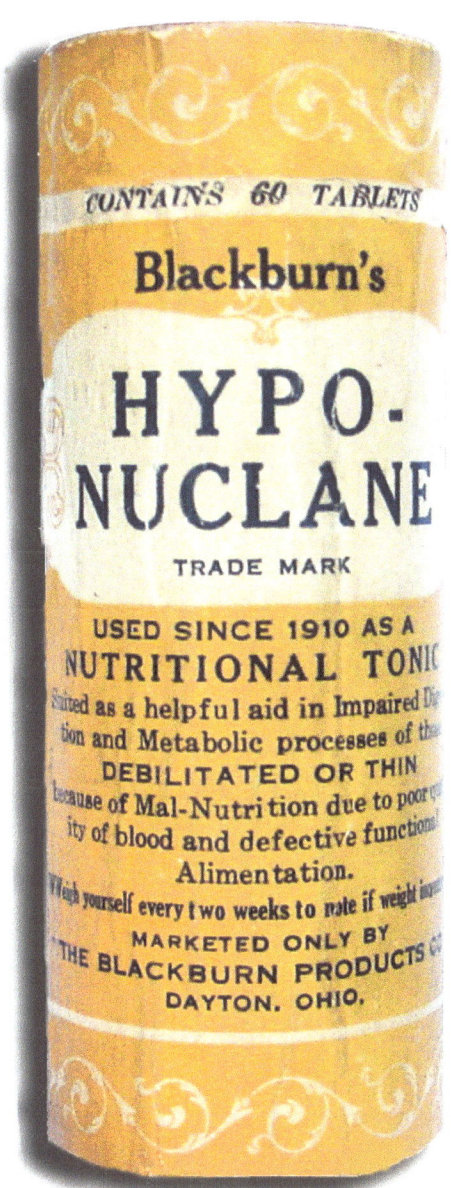

Advice on Beauty
by Claire Ainsworth

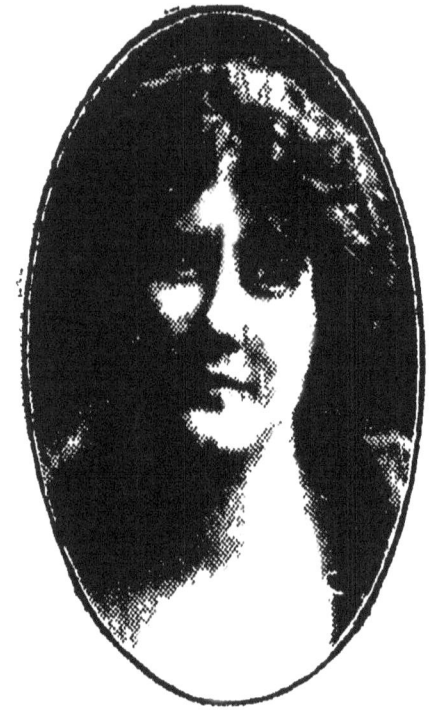

NOTE—If the reader does not find the information wanted in the questions answered below, just address a letter to Miss Claire Ainsworth, 40 Patterson Bldg., Dayton, Ohio, enclosing self-addressed stamped envelope, and she will gladly advise on health and beauty problems. The articles and preparations mentioned are on sale by all wholesale druggists, large retail and department stores, or any accommodating dealer can obtain them for you.

Answer to "Mabel R."—The best treatment that I know of to whiten a sallow skin and to remove pimples, blotches, etc., is a thorough course of one-grain quinoxide tablets. Get them of druggist in sealed tubes with full directions. Letters tell me that quinoxide always proves satisfactory.

Answer to "Maria R. C."—If your hair will not stay in curl and is straggling over the face and neck I would advise the regular use of wavolene. It is harmless, invisible, and keeps the hair in wave for days at a time, often causing a natural fluffy growth to ensue.

Answer to "Frances J."—A really fine hair tonic can be made by dissolving one-half ounce hairwand powder in a pint of soft water. It contains no alcohol which is harmful to the hair and hundreds of my correspondents are delighted with it.

Answer to "Mrs P. C."—I have frequently advised the taking of five-grain phythyrin tablets to reduce abnormal fatness and, judging from the many favorable and thankful letters I have received, this is the most effective and harmless remedy extant. These tablets are the result of exhaustive experiments conducted by physicians. After the first week or two reduction is usually rapid.

Answer to "Lucile B."—To remove hair growth in unnatural spots I advise the application of fluvol powder, which comes in sealed vials with directions for use. It is harmless and quickly removes the hair without marring the skin in any way.

Answer to "Mrs. B. G."—Dandruff is a loathsome disease of the scalp and if neglected causes ultimately the loss of the hair. A tried and proven remedy is plain yellow minyol, put up in four-ounce jars and widely used by professional hairdressers. Only a few applications are required, as a rule, and it greatly beautifies the hair.

Answer to "Augusta M."—I do know of a reliable massage to increase the bust and round the neck and arms. Apply regularly medicated venosol, and massage the parts as per directions with each sealed package and you will surely be delighted with the development which ensues. Many actresses have used it with benefit and loudly praise it as a true developer.

Answer to "M. G."—Always use a safe, harmless shampoo if you wish to improve your hair. Gloriol liquid shampoo is what I have used for years. Try it. I also use the gloriol face powder, deeming it superior to any other. Both are sold by druggists and at good toilet counters.

Answer to "Mrs C."—You can not gain flesh and become plump because you do not assimilate enough nourishment from the food you eat. Take three-grain hyponuclane tablets regularly and they will aid and improve your assimilative powers to such an extent that a very rapid gain should result. Some have gained as much as 40 pounds and their color and health are much better, too.

Answer to "Mary R."—A beautiful skin and complexion can be had by any one who will scientifically and regularly care for and properly massage the skin. I advise the use of pure, harmless creams. Gloriol emollient, gloriol balm, and gloriol glowene. Use them all, as per the directions, they are inexpensive and reliable, and never fail to produce very fine skin and complexion, if used regularly and intelligently. Space will not permit me to give methods of massage, but I will gladly send you or anyone my book, "Beauty Truths," upon receipt of two stamps. This book is worth many dollars, but for a short time I will send it free.—Advertisement.

Claire Ainswoth's column ran from 1912 to 1915. Although reported to be a well-known singer, her name does not appear in any census records from 1900 to 1920, nor in the Dayton city directory from 1900 to 1925.

Weight Loss

Even a century ago women were concerned with being thin. It was the fashion to wear slender dresses not really made for the average size woman. Blackburn's answer to weight loss was "Phythyrin Tablets." The result of "exhaustive experiments conducted by physicians" the tablets were used to reduce abnormal fatness without the need to diet or exercise. In her column, Claire would write of how easy it was for obese people to lose weight. In fact, "it is such a simple matter in this day and age to reduce excessive fatness that I wonder why there are any such." She guaranteed that using Phythyrin Tablets would reduce anyone "surely and steadily."

Bust Enlargers

It seems that many of Claire Ainsworth's readers would write in complaining of being "terribly flat-chested and having no bust development at all." One letter writer almost begged for advice on how to "overcome this unnatural condition." Claire endorsed a cream made by the Blackburn Company called "Medicated Venosol" that, if used religiously, would reward the user with a "well-developed bust." For those who wrote in wondering if they were wrong to worry about their "physical state", Claire explained of how it was normal to crave a "natural form and figure which lends so much to a woman's beauty and magnetism."

> *It is the duty of every girl and woman to always appear at her best...It is not vanity that impels you to seek; it is good common sense. Many actresses and society women indorse this treatment.*

The cream was to be rubbed into the skin for ten minutes or more at least two or three times a day. One claim made was that a user went from a size 30 to a size 38 chest in only three months.

Blackburn Products wasn't the only Dayton company to promote a bust developing cream. In 1907 The Globe Pharmaceutical Company began marketing what was known as "Sartoin Skin Food." The company modestly claimed that their preparation "is probably the most effective remedy known to science for sunburn, rashes and all skin blemishes" and that it was equally effective in "creating the normal growth of all parts not fully developed and shrunken" or, in other words, a bust developer.

The Bureau of Chemistry analyzed a sample of the "skin food" and found that "the most effective remedy known to science" was essentially Epsom salts colored with a pink dye. The government frowned on the company claiming Epsom salts to be a food. William E. Pilkinton and A. P. Foose, owners of the Globe Pharmaceutical Company, were charged with selling a product whose claims were false, misleading and deceptive. The men pled guilty and were each fined $10.

PRESCRIPTION FOR COMPLEXION AND SKIN FOOD MIXTURE.

The formula given below is said to be the most effective known to science for clearing the complexion and developing shrunken or hollow parts It is in general use among the French society women, who are renowned all over the world for their exquisite complexions Procure from the druggist the following

Two ounces of Rose Water one ounce Spirits of Cologne four ounces Sartoin (crystallized)

Put the Sartoin into a pint of hot water (not boiling) and when dissolved and cooled strain through a fine cloth then add the Rose Water and Cologne Spirits

This is to be applied daily to the face neck and bust and massage thoroughly into the skin If the treatment is persistently used remarkable results will follow even for the worst complexion or roughest skin The above formula is inexpensive and makes sufficient of the mixture to last a month.

M. D. COURCEY'S
HAIR TONIC,
For Promoting the Growth of the Hair,
MANUFACTURED AND FOR SALE BY
M. D. COURCEY,
Cor. Jefferson and Market streets,
DAYTON, OHIO.

IT is peculiarly adapted for the use of Ladies, as it will without fail, promote the growth of the hair, and unlike a great many of the so-called Hair Tonics, will restore and not injure the hair.
je27

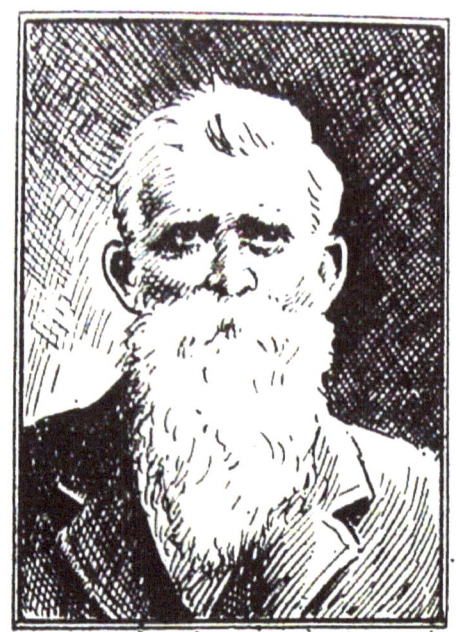

THE NEW WONDER!

Peter Josse's Hair Restorative!

THIS Hair Restorative is now acknowledged to be the best ever invented for all diseases of the Hair and the Scalp, and it has worked wonders wherever used. Several of our citizens have tried it, and speak in the highest terms of its curative properties. The following is one among the many certificates just received by the Proprietor:—

DAYTON, Sept. 9th, 1859.

MR. P. JOSSE:—For several years past, from some cause, our hair has been gradually falling out, until entire baldness threatened us. We have tried various remedies, but without any good result. We were induced to try your "Restorative" by hearing it highly spoken of by those who had used it, and who assured us that it had the effect of bringing a new and vigorous growth of hair upon their heads. We have used it, and its good effects are plainly visible in the renewed growth of hair where we were fast becoming bald. We cannot recommend the Restorative too highly.

Yours, truly,
WM. SWALEM,
S. L. BROADWELL,
OWEN TRENOR,
J. J. SWALEM.

For sale at the Barber Shop of Peter Josse, 41, Jefferson street, Dayton. sept16-3wd

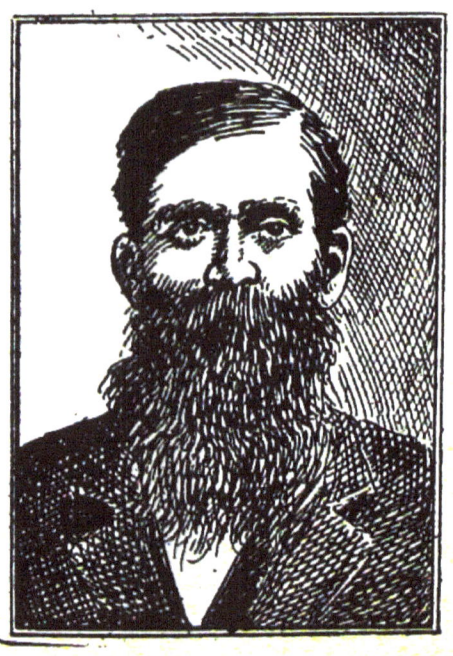

Men had their own issues when it came to looking their best. In 1859 men from the Gem City turned to M. D. Courcey and Peter Josse for help in growing new hair on balding heads.

In 1910 John W. Hefferline began selling a hair-tonic and hair restorer that supposedly not only made hair grow but also brought back its natural color. The trademark for the nostrum used drawings of Hefferline, (above) presumably before and after he used his hair restorer. In 1912 Hefferline was granted Trademark Patent #63,729 for his self-portraits.

Chapter Fourteen
Testimonials

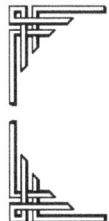
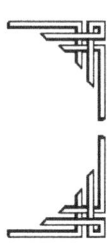

How could the same people who did not trust their doctors turn around and be persuaded to trust their health to a perfect stranger? Much of this came from the use of what was known as a "testimonial", where an individual would claim to have been helped or cured by a particular nostrum. Testimonials were the bread and butter of the patent medicine manufacturers. Used as advertisements in newspapers, almanacs and trade cards, a sincere testimonial brought more customers. Although some testimonials were completely made up, others were written by buyers who really believed they had benefited from the product.

Many patent medicine firms claimed that they had thousands of unsolicited testimonials on how well their product worked. The fact of the matter was that most of the testimonials were worthless. An article by George Frank Lord, on "Testimonials in Advertising" (*Printer's Ink*, February 3, 1909), wrote that, although the testimonials were usually genuine, "the average patent medicine ad appeals chiefly to hypochondriacs who are not sick, but imagine they are when they read their 'symptoms.' The same ad creates the sickness and effects a cure..."

Most illnesses usually last only a short period of time. If the disease is not chronic or fatal, the human body will usually cure itself if left alone. Nostrum manufacturers understood this and used it to sell their products. They also knew that even chronic diseases run in stages. A person looking for relief would of course not be feeling well. Most times the person would feel better after taking the medication, at least for a short while, which would have happened anyway.

Some of the testimonials used were "enhanced" from information the companies received from users of their products. In the New York Tribune for March 12, 1916, Samuel Hopkins Adams wrote an article titled "How Testimonials Are Faked for Nostrums; Valueless Endorsements Made from Little or Nothing Without Users' Consent." The nostrum Mr. Adams focused on was Tanlac, at the time being made by the Cooper Medicine Company in Dayton. Part of the article is reprinted here:

How Testimonials Are Faked for Nostrums
by Samuel Hopkins Adams

Medical testimonials are generally recognized as the flimsiest sort of evidence. About 99 per cent of them emanate from persons too ignorant to understand the nature of the disease or the process of recovery. Often they are paid for. Not infrequently they receive a posthumous publication, the writer, after producing his or her endorsement, having promptly died of the very disease which the patent medicine has so convincingly cured - in print...

Discredited though the patent-medicine testimonials are for general character, it is seldom that [a view of] the specific internal process of the lie-factories which turn them out wholesale is afforded. This kind of work is usually done behind closed doors. By a happy chance, I am enabled to give here a public view of the very private enterprise of faking a testimonial... The nostrum caught in the act is Tanlac.

Tanlac is supposed to be a marvelous and mysterious 'discovery', and a sort of cure-all for people who are out of sorts... From its alcohol it derives the 'kick' which enables it to pose as a tonic, and by its testimonials it inspires the confidence of the weak-minded upon whom it depends for its sales.

Had its advertising been only just good enough to impress the weak-minded alone, this article would never have been written. Unfortunately for it, one of its lures in print so skillfully set forth its claims that it arrested the attention of Mrs. V. W. Tripler (this is not her correct name, as she is adverse to further publicity), of Chattanooga, Tenn., who is by no means weak-minded. In fact, Mrs. Tripler is not at all the stuff which good, paying, convincing unreliable testimonials are made, and the local Tanlac man committed his fatal error in assuming that she was. His name is Warren, and he is stationed at the Live & Let Live Drug Store and testimonial sub-station, of Chattanooga. It was he who, adding his persuasions to the advertising of Tanlac, induced Mrs. Tripler to buy six bottles of the preparation, to cure her of a slight nervousness from which she was suffering. Being a business woman, Mrs. Tripler thought that she should receive a discount for quantity. Warren consented to give her six bottles for $5 provided that she would furnish a testimonial for the medicine. This she agreed to do in case she was benefited by Tanlac.

Less than two bottles of the marvelous discovery had been taken by Mrs. Tripler when Warren appeared at the office of which Mr. Tripler is proprietor, with a testimonial form-blank all ready for the statement and signature of Mrs. Tripler, who assists her husband in his work. The form was a catechism of ills and aches and ailments. The witness to the virtues of Tanlac was requested to state whether she had suffered from an appalling variety of symptoms, sicknesses, and habits, of which constipation, indigestion, insomnia and biliousness are mild examples. Mrs. Tripler not having the testimonial habit, answered 'No' to nearly everything. All that was wrong with her, she explained to Warren, was nervousness, and not much of that. Mr. Tripler objected to her giving any testimonial at all, believing that the medicine was worthless; but his wife felt that she was in honor bound to give some return for her discount, so her husband typed in her replies on his typewriter. When it was all done Warren looked it over and ruefully observed that nobody could make much of a testimonial out of that. Therein he did himself and the Tanlac Company less than justice. For, a few days later, after it had been through his hands and those of G. F. Willis, the testimonial expert of the concern, it blossomed forth in the Chattanooga News in a form which caused the Triplers more surprise than gratification. Some of the reasons why [they were] not inspired to paeans of rejoicing may be discovered in the parallel herewith furnished of the testimonial as revised by a treatment of Tanlac, and the actual facts concerning Mrs. Tripler.

[Statements from the Tanlac article are in italics, the facts stated by Mr. And Mrs. Tripler to Samuel Hopkins Adams are in bold print. - Editor]

"I had been in wretched health for a long time," said Mrs. Tripler, "and I was just about on the verge of a nervous breakdown when I found Tanlac."
Mrs. Tripler had not been in wretched health, either for a long time or a short time, and did not consider herself on the verge of a nervous breakdown.

"I was so run down and debilitated that I couldn't even stand for the children to be around me, and almost everything irritated me and made me miserable."
One possible reason for her inability to endure 'the presence of the children" is that she has no children. They are the off-spring of the Tanlac testimonial-faker's fervid fancy.

"I couldn't sleep at night and I got so bad I would have shaking spells. After having these nervous attacks I would feel weal all over and tremble like a leaf."
At no time has Mrs. Tripler suffered from sleeplessness. This she specifically stated to Warren. The shaking spells were provided for her through the courtesy of Tanlac; and the nervous attacks when she "would feel weak all over and would tremble like a leaf." She never experienced any such symptoms in her own person. Tanlac invented them and "wished them" on her.

"My digestion was bad, and I was bilious and constipated and had no appetite."
If her digestion was bad, Tanlac must have made it so, for there had never been anything wrong with it previous to Warren's call, as she carefully informed him. She was neither bilious nor constipated, and her appetite was good.

"I had no energy and the smallest task about the house would exhaust me completely... That dreadful nervous condition has entirely disappeared and I can go about my household duties with my old energy and lightheartedness."

Among her friends Mrs. Tripler has always been regarded as a woman of exceptional energy and activity, a "live wire." The household duties, which are supposed to have wearied her so until Tanlac made them light, are, like the children, figments of the Tanlac fake factory. Mrs. Tripler does nothing whatever in the line of household duties, but spends her entire day at her husband's plant, assisting him.

Commenting on this case, Mr. G. F. Willis, Southern distributor of Tanlac said: "I am quite certain I understand Mrs. Tripler's condition."

He ought to! He wrote it.

There, in its entirety, is how patent medicine testimonials are manufactured, when they are not bought outright or beguiled by treachery from the ignorant and unreasoning. The whole testimonial industry is tainted with fraud and deceit. Before you yield to temptation to buy a nostrum on the strength of some indorsement or other, Stop! Look! Listen! It may have been treated with Tanlac.

"IT CERTAINLY HAS HELPED ME" SAYS MRS. TRIPLER

Chattanooga Woman Faced a Nervous Breakdown

Was So Nervous She Would Shake Like a Leaf

Tanlac Readily Overcomes Trouble After All Other Medicines Failed

Hundreds of Chattanooga people, both men and women, have taken Tanlac with the most astonishing and gratifying results, and during recent weeks the number has increased so rapidly that there is seldom a day that a number of remarkable reports from relieved sufferers do not find their way to the Live & Let Live Drug Store.

Mrs. Tripler, wife of the proprietor of a well known [business] in this city, is still another who has cause to be glad she has heard of this great medicine.

Facsimile used by Samuel Hopkins Adams to illustrate the fake testimonial put out by the Live and Let Live Drug Store *that appeared in the Chattanooga* News. *Adams did not use the original Tanlac advertisement in his article so that the real identity of "Mrs. Tripler" would remain a secret.*

When Samuel Hopkins Adams mentions in his article that some of the writers of the testimonials "receive a posthumous publication...having promptly died of the very disease which the patent medicine has so convincingly cured," he wasn't kidding. On March 15, 1918 a testimonial appeared in the *Cumberland Evening Times* of how Alfred L. Wingert had suffered for years with pains in the stomach and even had to retire from work because of ill health. Luckily, he sent for a bottle of Tanlac. "Tanlac has done me a wonderful lot of good," Wingert wrote after he had begun using the medicine. "My health is surely coming back to me."

Well, not quite. It seems that Wingert had actually died on March 9th, a week before his testimonial appeared in the paper, from chronic interstitial nephritis; a kidney disorder of which among its symptoms are nausea and vomiting.

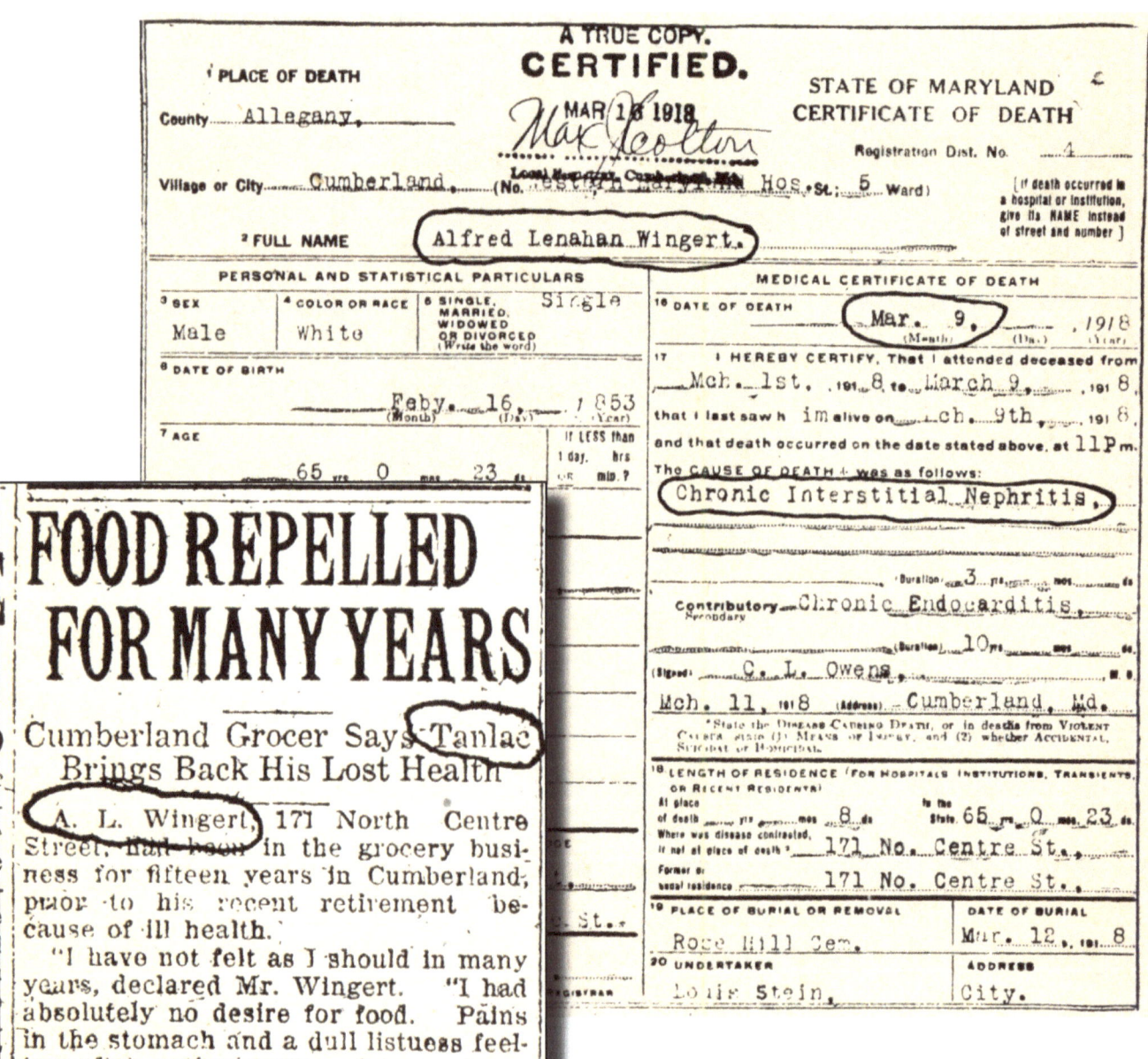

Alfred Lenahan Wingert had been dead nearly a week when his testimonial appeared in the newspaper. He had just turned 65 years old less than a month before.

THREE IN ONE FAMILY MAKES UNUSUAL CASE

South Hadley Falls Man Relieved of Stomach Trouble Since Taking Tanlac, the National Tonic.

"I HAVE GAINED 10 POUNDS"

Says Fred Wicks, "and My Wife and Son Are Also Taking Tanlac and Have Been Greatly Benefited."

Health is wealth. Health is the greatest wealth in the world—the soundest capital, the biggest asset. Without health the bloated bond holder is a pauper. With health the plodding laborer is rich. All the money in the world cannot buy this asset of health that is absolutely necessary for success of any kind. The man without health is beaten before he begins his fight. He does not even qualify for a trial. He is barred from ever trying. Mr. Fred Wicks of 52 Granby Road, South Hadley Falls, Mass., has been relieved of stomach trouble and has gained 10 pounds in weight since taking Tanlac. His wife and son are also tak-

FUNERALS

WICK—The funeral of Fred Wick was held this morning from his home, Granby Road, South Hadley Falls, followed by a high mass of requiem in St. Patrick's church. Rev. J. E. Sellig officiated. The bearers were Jacob and John Miller, Charles Todt, Charles P. O'Connor, John St. John and James Kelly. The burial was held in the St. Jerome cemetery.

On May 11, 1917 Fred Wick's testimonial appeared in a Tanlac ad in the Holyoke Daily Transcript. In it Wick states that, after taking the medication, he no longer suffered from stomach problems and had in fact gained ten pounds. In the same issue of the newspaper, under the bold heading of "Funerals", appeared the notice that 'the funeral of Fred Wick was held this morning…" Wick's death certificate showed that he had died of cancer of the stomach *two days before his testimonial was published.*

Chapter Fifteen
The Art of Advertising

In 1891 Lee J. Vance wrote an article for *Popular Science Monthly*, stating how important advertising was to the patent medicine industry.

> *Frankly speaking, nostrum vendors no longer rely on the curative powers of their drugs. They depend now on the power of advertising exclusively. They have a literary man to "write up" the remedy in ingenious fashion; an artist to show the patient "before and after" using the panacea; a poet to compose odes and lyrics; a liar who rivals Munchhausen; and a forger who signs all kinds of testimonials.*

Even though there was evidence that people were dying in spite of taking patent medicines, or perhaps because of it, many newspapers did not report it. In fact, not only did the newspapers modify news that might harm nostrum manufacturers, in some cases they helped fight legislature that might have put the medicine makers out of business.

The Civil War helped the medicine sellers in a subtle, but substantial, way. People couldn't get enough news about the war. Weekly newspapers became dailies and circulation increased. After the war was over and circulation dropped, newspapers came to depend on their advertising dollars to keep afloat. In many cases their biggest advertisers were patent medicine companies.

The remedy sellers were quick to realize this. They used the situation as a way to begin controlling what the newspapers said. The companies would sign two or three year contracts with a newspaper, agreeing to buy a certain amount of advertising during that period of time. As a precaution, however, the contracts would also include what would become known as the "red letter" clause.

Legend states that F. J. Cheney, the proprietor of Hall's Catarrh Cure, was the first to include the clause in his deals. Every advertising contract he

Advertising contract containing the "red letter" clause.

made with the newspapers had printed on it, in bold red letters, "It is mutually agreed that this Contract is void if any law is enacted by your State restricting or prohibiting the manufacture or sale of proprietary medicine." This, of course, put the newspapers in a bind, almost forcing them to put the patent medicine sellers in as good a light as possible. Whenever a piece of legislature threatened the medicine company's profit margin, letters would be sent out to the various newspapers reminding them of the clause. This usually resulted in the papers endorsing their advertiser's position, both in print and in letters to their local and state representatives. If a newspaper took the position of not defending the medicine manufacturers, it took the risk of losing all of its advertising from that source, which could cause some damage. As late as 1898 medicines and remedies still accounted for more than twice as much advertising than any other class of product. Competition in the proprietary medicine business was fierce, with some companies spending 30 to 40 percent of the gross sales in advertising their products. The Dr. Harter Medicine Company reportedly spent over a half-million dollars each year in advertising.

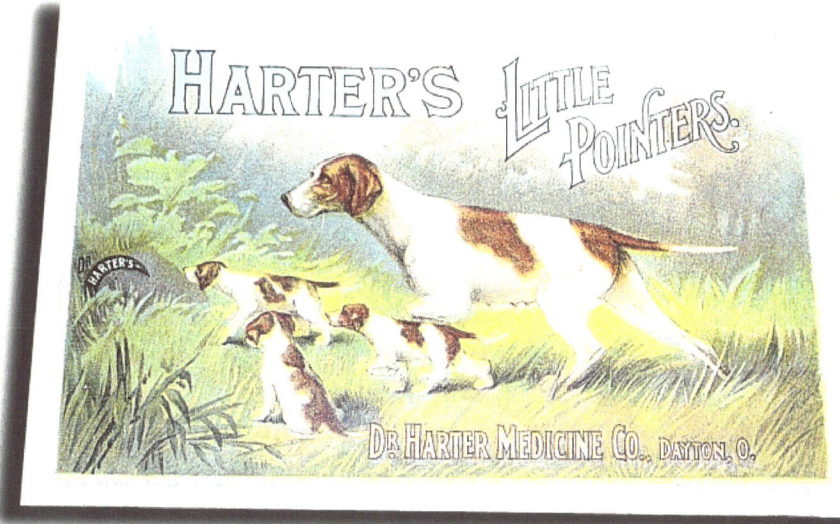

   Of course, nostrum sellers didn't just rely on newspapers for promoting their merchandise. Almanacs were devoted to weather information, advice on planting, phases of the moon, and an annual calendar. At first patent medicine companies ran ads in regular almanacs. then bought them and gave them away. Eventually the larger medicine makers began printing out their own almanacs, devoting the ads to their firm alone. The companies sometimes walked a fine line trying to figure out how many ads could be added to the almanac, while still making it useful and entertaining enough to keep through the season.

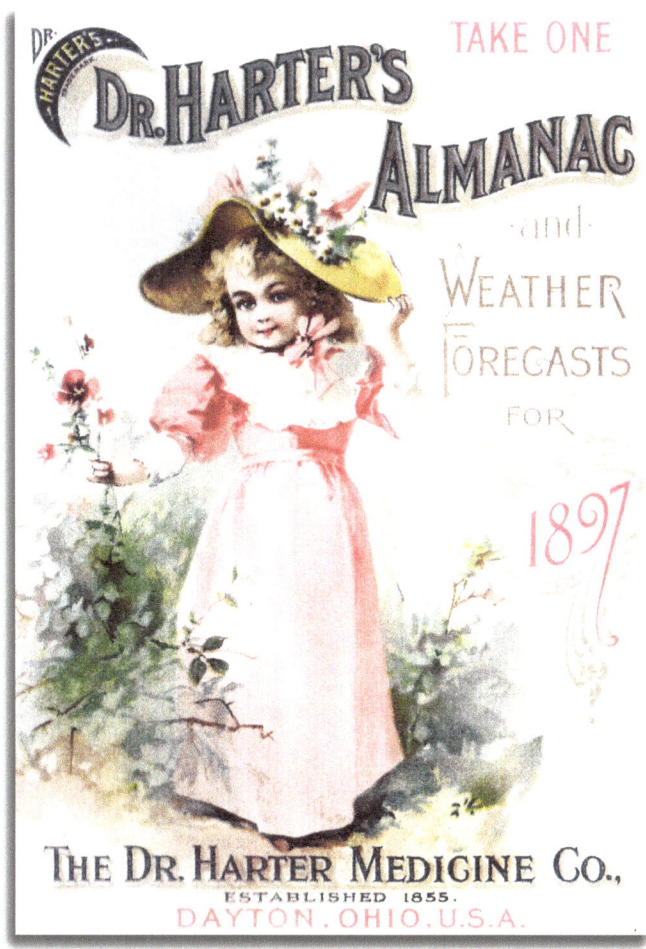
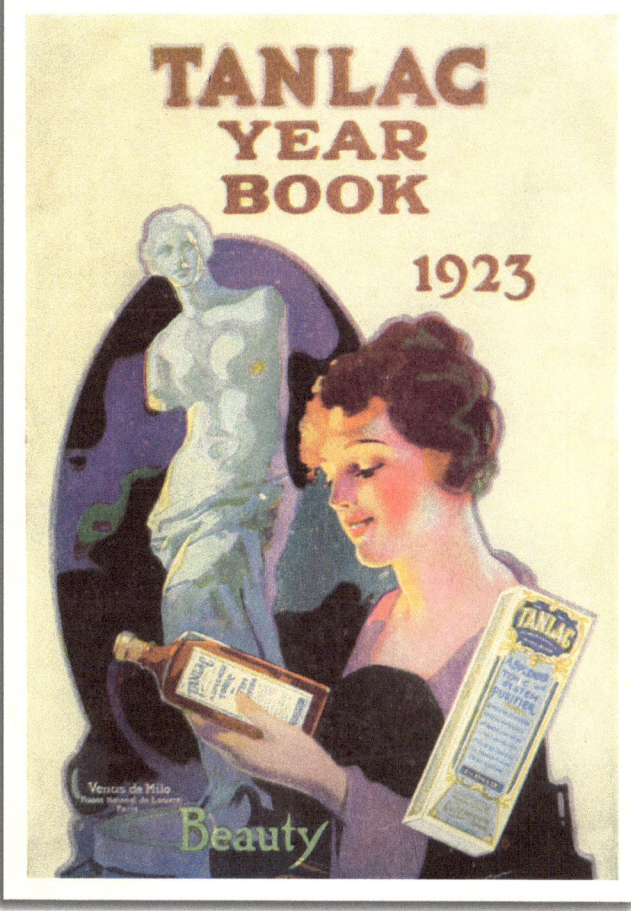

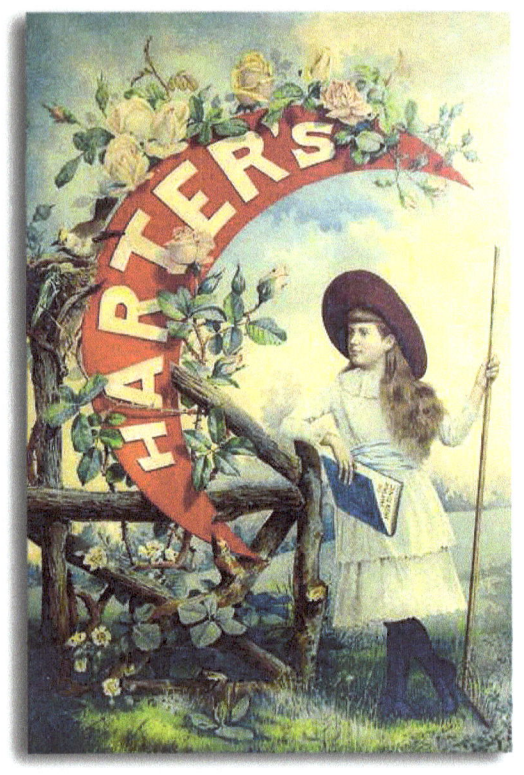 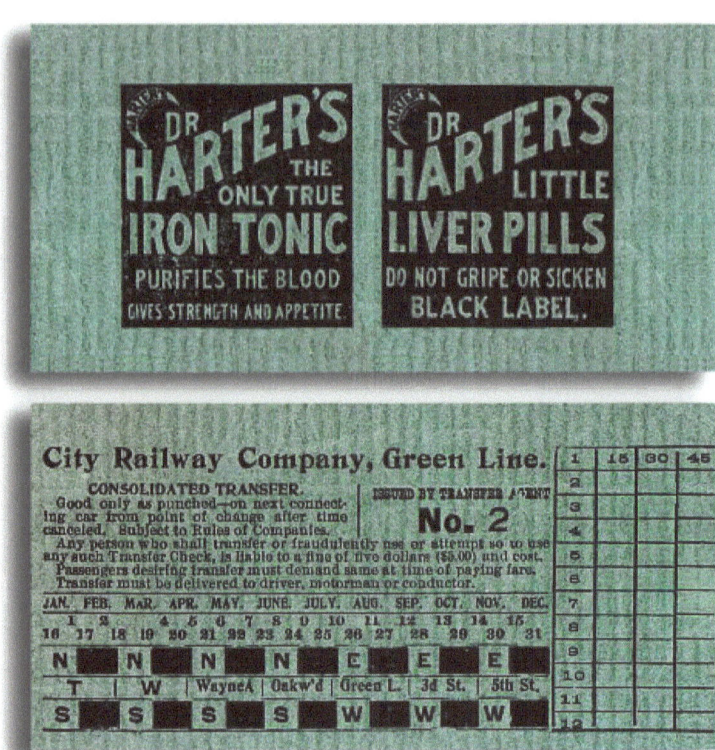

When the Dr. Harter Medicine Company opened their new building in Dayton in 1895, over 10,000 feet of floor space was entirely devoted to a vast printing department which was used to print a number of advertising items.

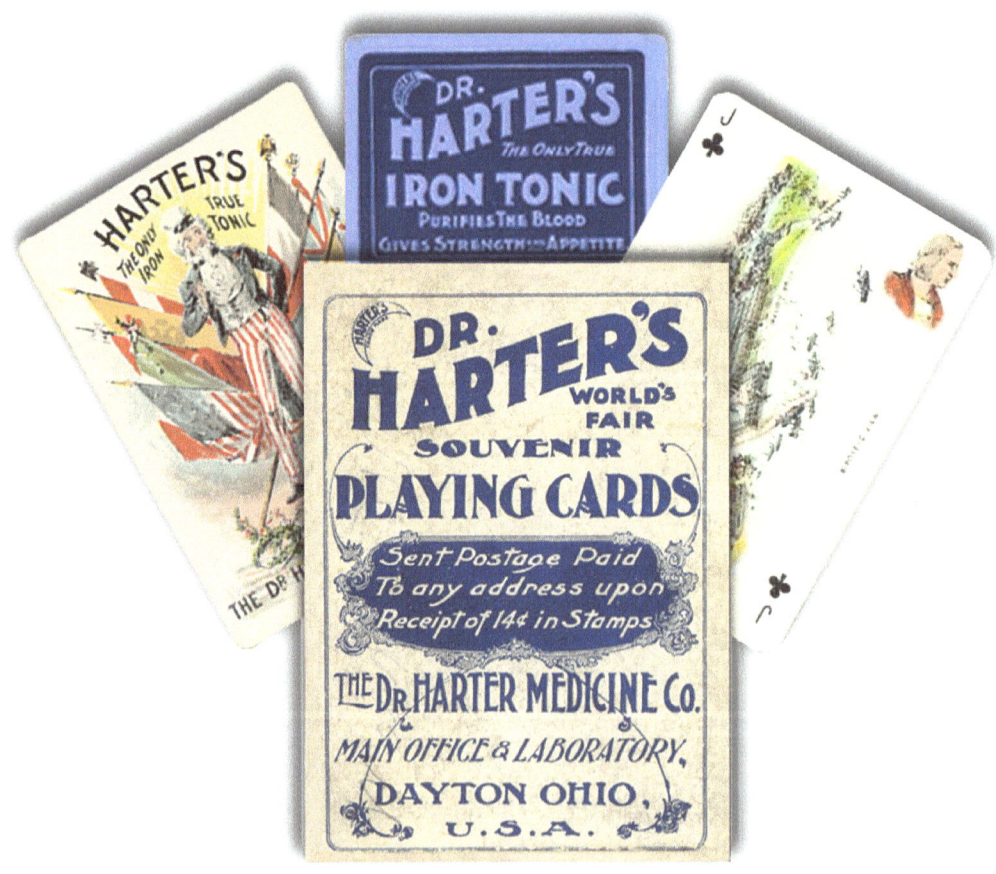

Dr. Oliver Crook & Company went so far as to enter the publishing field in order to get their message across. In 1868 the company published the novel *The Nautch Girl!* by Washington Chanter. The book was printed in serial form, with parts of the novel coming out each week for twelve weeks. At the interesting parts of the story an ad or testimonial for Crook's Wine of Tar would appear. The sections were free to anyone who asked, but were only available in drugs stores that sold Dr. Crook's medicines.

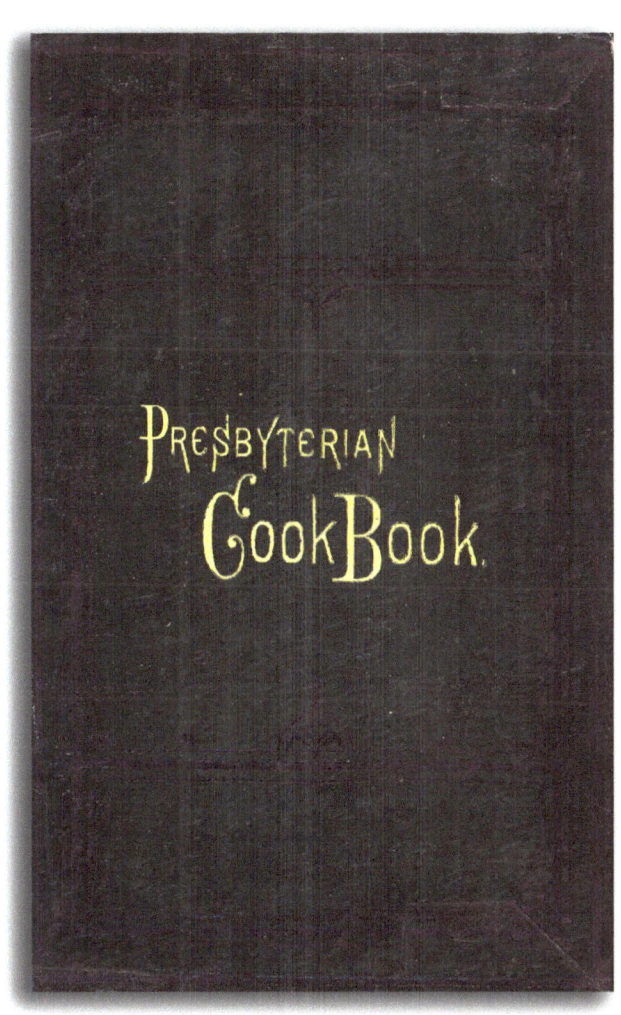

In 1872 the company was also responsible for printing the *Presbyterian Cookbook*, which contained a number of recipes that had been compiled by members of the First Presbyterian Church in Dayton, Ohio. A small ad for Dr. Crook's Wine of Tar was placed in the back of the cookbook.

Patent medicine companies were also among the first to use trade cards on a wide scale. Trade cards gave the patent medicine companies a certain freedom from restraints that would have been imposed by some of the periodical publications. The cards allowed the advertised to make whatever claims they wished, no matter how fantastic those statements might be. Many times the cards would list a seemingly unending supply of ailments that would be cured by the medicine, some even claiming their product was helpful in treating the ills of both humans and animals.

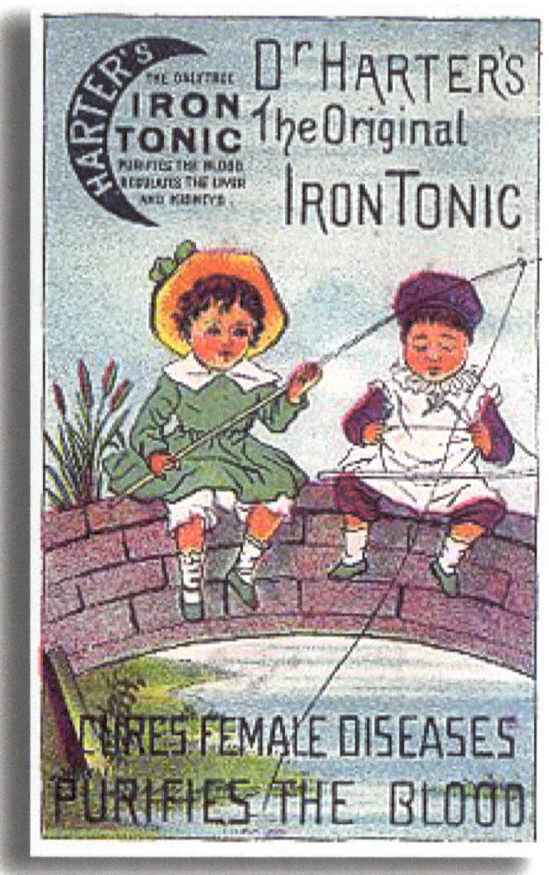

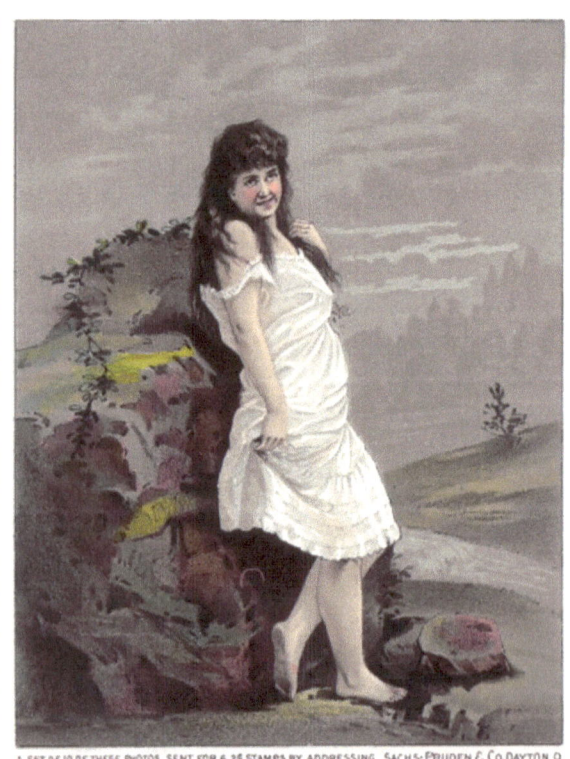

Chapter Sixteen
The Decline of Patent Medicines

In the later decades of the nineteenth century journalists began writing exposés on patent medicine companies, stating how worthless or dangerous some of the products were. Samuel Hopkins Adams wrote the most famous series of articles on patent medicine. Entitled *The Great American Fraud*, the series ran in the *Collier's Weekly* magazine from October 1905 to February 1906. His articles attacked patent medicine makers and their co-conspirators in the press who refused to investigate the truth of the ads they were printing. He criticized nostrum manufacturers and told of how the companies would trade mailing lists of people who sent in personal letters of medical inquiry. These unsuspecting sufferers would then be bombarded with letters from various medicine makers who unerringly seemed to know what aliment they suffered from and, luckily, also sold something to cure it.

In 1906 the American Medical Association set up a laboratory to evaluate which medicines were creditable enough to be granted permission to advertise in the AMA *Journal*. This led to the creation of a Propaganda Department that gathered information concerning health fraud and quack products. In 1911 the AMA published their findings in a book entitled *Nostrums and Quackery*, which was later expanded into three volumes.

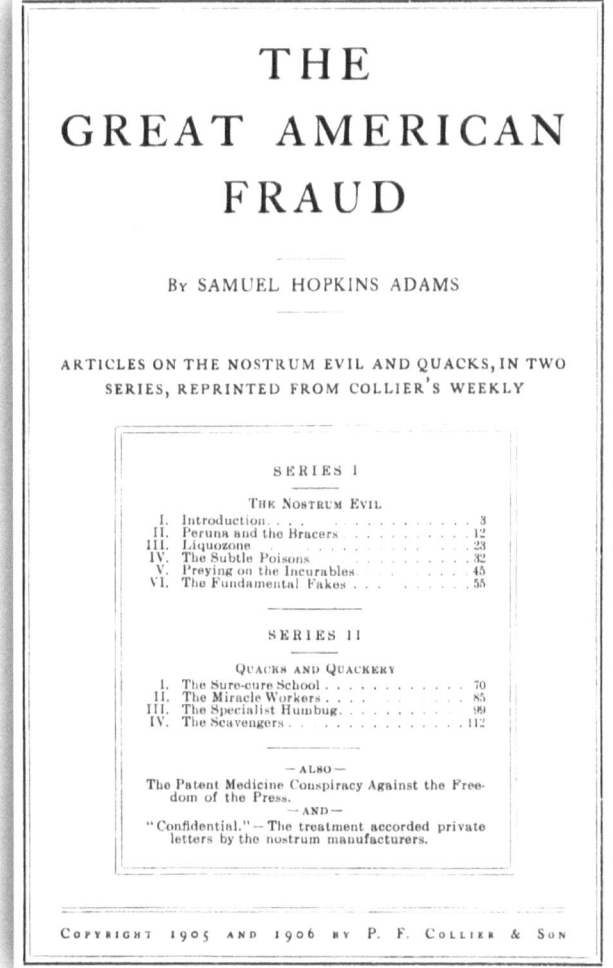

In 1905 Samuel Hopkins Adams wrote a series of eleven articles for Collier's Weekly exposing many of the false statements made by patent medicine manufacturers about their products, as well as pointing out that in some instances the medicines were actually harmful. In 1906 the American Medical Association reprinted Adams' series in book form, which eventually sold over a half-million copies.

At the time, the federal government was not responsible for the quality of food and drugs in the United States. The responsibility for the safety of locally made drugs generally fell on the individual states. Adams' articles so outraged the public that they began pressuring federal officials to set more secure rules on what food and drugs contained. This led to the Pure Food and Drugs Act, which was signed into law on June 30, 1906. The act prohibited the interstate transport of unlawful and mislabeled food and drugs. Manufacturers were required to list the presence and amount of certain dangerous ingredients including alcohol, heroin, and cocaine on their drug labels. Any ingredient not considered dangerous did not have to be listed, but if it was on the label, then the product had to contain it.

This did not close all the loopholes, but it was a beginning. The Sherley Amendment in 1912 prohibited misleading statements on labels. It was this amendment that forced medicine manufacturers to start using the word "remedy" instead of "cure" on their labels. The Durham-Humphrey Act of 1951 increased the control of certain drugs, defining the types of drugs that could not be safely used without medical supervision and restricted their sale to prescription by a licensed practitioner. In 1962 the Kefauver-Harris Amendment required drug manufacturers to prove to the FDA the effectiveness of their products before selling them.

As each amendment was passed, the number of patent medicines on the market declined. This does not mean, however, that they are completely gone. Most drug stores still sell products that are almost completely useless. Today's modern patent medicines include a wide range of items, from certain vitamins and herbs, to fat-burning and sexual enhancing pills that vaguely promise to help improve the quality of the buyer's life. And, just as it was a century ago, advertisers still play on people's desires and fears to make money from products that may do more harm than good.

For example: On July 24, 2003, Congress launched an investigation of a dietary supplement called ephedra to determine if it had caused the death of over 100 users. By this time ephedra had been bought by thousands of people, the supplement being especially popular among young people seeking to lose weight or build muscle. Unlike drugs, dietary supplements did not have to be proven safe before going on the market.

On October 25, 1994 the Dietary Supplement Health and Education Act of 1994 (DSHEA) was passed. FDA began regulating dietary supplements under a different set of rules than those covering "conventional" foods and prescription and over-the-counter drugs. Under DSHEA the dietary supplement manufacturer became responsible for ensuring that a dietary supplement was safe before being marketed. Generally, manufacturers did not need to register their products with the FDA or get FDA approval before producing or selling dietary supplements. It was up to the manufacturers to make sure that product label information was truthful and not misleading.

During the hearings Representative John D. Dingell spoke of how legal loopholes had weakened the intent of the act.

(T)he law cannot be used to adequately protect the public from these modern day patent medicine peddlers and snake oil salesmen. Given the state of law, at least as currently interpreted, there is simply no way that even educated consumers can distinguish between dietary supplements that can provide real benefit at an affordable price and often dangerous rip-offs that have become pervasive, at least amongst the heavily advertised products of this industry. I will point out that this industry is full of shysters, they are not properly required to label the products or to be regulated as to either safety, efficacy or the quality of manufacturing practices... American consumers deserve to be able to get vitamins and other supplements that will enhance their lives without falling prey to charlatans and scoundrels that promise the impossible but not only deliver disappoint at best, but disaster at worst.

On February 12, 2004 the FDA announced that the sale of dietary supplements containing ephedrine alkaloids was prohibited, since such supplements presented an unreasonable risk of illness or injury.

As long as man wants to lose weight without exercise or cure whatever ails him without having to work for it, there will be someone out there willing to con them out of their money.

Patent Medicine Sellers in Dayton 1858-1933

From 1858 to 1933 over 200 companies and individuals began advertising in Dayton city directories as sellers or manufacturers of patent medicines. This included agents representing proprietary manufacturers not from Dayton. This distinction was often not made in the directories. Also, an individual may have been in business for several years prior to, or for several years after, thier advertising started or stopped in the city directories. The symbol * after a name indicates there is more information at the bottom of the same page on that particular seller that was not listed in previous chapters in this book.

Albert Chemical Co., The (1931-1934)
418 McLain	1931
436 Wayne Ave.	1932-34

Allen, Robert W. (1890-1896)
827 South Brown	1890-91
232 East Xenia Ave.	1891-92
806 East Xenia Ave.	1894-95
309 West 3rd	1895-96

American Drug Co. (1918-1922)
4th floor 24 North Jefferson	1918-22

American Herb Medicine Co. (1888-1892)*
422 East 5th	1888-91
swc 5th and Stone	1892

Ampula, Boleshaw (1922-1932)
912 North Valley	1922-32

Ankenbrock, John (1908-1910)
1151 West 3rd	1908-10

Anzer, Joseph (1902-1906)
141 East 5th	1902-06

Approved Formula Co., The (1911-1913)
nec 1st and Canal	1911-13

Arnold Laboratories Co., The (1921)
nec 2nd and Main, room 35	1921

Arras, Anna E. (1874-1890)
5 Webster, btwn 1st & 2nd	1874-83
39 South VanLear	1884-90

Austin, Waterman (1871-74)**
16 McLane	1871-74

Bailey & Franklin (1889-91)
745 West Washington, Patterson	1889-91

Bailey, Jesse A. (1892-10)
745 West Washington, Patterson	1892-10

Banus Remedy Co. (1902-36)
314 East Xenia Ave.	1913-17
625 East Xenia Ave.	1918-21
1559 East Richard	1922-24
625 East Xenia Ave.	1925-27
22 Park Ave.	1928-36

Barber Remedey Co. (1902)
316 S. Warren	1902

Beard, F. Co. (1903-05, 1908)
238 N. McDaniel	1903-04
784 West River	1904-05
266 West River	1908

Bentley, George F. (1908)
49 South Bonner	1908

Binkley, J. C. (1903-04)
46 East 2nd	1903-04

Binkley, J. Z. (1904-09)
106 West 5th	1904-06
46 East 2nd	1907-08
204 South Ludlow	1908-09

Binkley, J. Z. & Son (1909-10)
204 South Ludlow	1909-10

Blackburn Products Co., The (1908-47)
nec 5th and Summit	1908-09
312 South College	1909-42
1652 Brown	1943-47

Bliss Native Herbs (1914-16)**
64 South Horton	1914-16

Bliss, The Alonzo O. Co. (1900-01)**
141 East 5th	1900-01

BLK Medicine Co. (1923-27)
room 26, 38 East 5th	1923-27

---

*   The American Herb Medicine Company was out of Washington D.C.
** Waterman Austin is listed in 1874 as manufacturing "Indian Salve"
*** Both Bliss Native Herbs and The Alonzo O. Bliss Co. was out of Washington, D.C.

Blondheim, Julius (1923)
   249 Samuel   1923

Blue Grass Chemical Co. (1925-30)
   1028 Washington   1925-26
   959 Washington   1929-30

Boen, Zaza M. (1932-37)
   1218 East Herman Ave.   1932-33
   40 High   1933-37

Bolender, John (1902-04)
   408 S. Hopeland   1902-04

Bowanee Medicine Co. (1889-95)
   138 North Canal   1889-90
   115 North Sears   1890-91
   113 North Sears   1893-95

Brace Specialty Co. (1908)
   65 South LaBelle   1908

Brandon Medicine Co., The (1891-94)*
   swc 4th   1891-93
   room A, Kuhns Bldg.   1893-94
   19 Davies Bldg.   1894

Brennert, Carl H. (1927-34)
   314 Xenia Ave.   1927-34

Brown, Catherine (1875-77)**
   401 Howard   1875-77

Brown, Martha (1908-10)
   919 East 5th   1908-10

Bucher, Henry J. (1915)
   1016 West 3rd   1915

Buckeye Medicine Co. (1900-04)***
   612 East 1st   1900-04

Burge-Layton Inc. (1924-36)
   nec 2nd and Main   1924
   510 Wayne Ave.   1925-36

Cain, Dennis (1886-96)
   122 North Troy   1886-96

Coffin, Erastus (1876-77)
   37 Richard   1876-77
   110 Miami   1877

Cole, Benjamin F. (1889-96)
   447 West 3rd   1889-90
   582 West 3rd   1891-92
   805 East 5th   1892-93
   603 East 5th   1893-95
   1204 East 5th   1895-96

Continental Specialty Co. (1909-11)
   132 East 2nd   1909-11

Cooper Laboatories Inc. (1928-29)
   nec 2nd and Main   1928
   301 East 1st   1929

Cooper Medicine Co., The (1902-24)
   812 East 5th   1902-03
   113 East 2nd   1903-05
   nec 1st and Canal   1906-13
   2nd floor 309 East 1st   1914-24

Cooper, J. L. (1924)
   416 nec 2nd and Main   1924

Creighton, Thomas (1877)
   sec 3rd and Jefferson   1877

Crook, Oliver & Co. (1868-74)
   239 1/2 3rd   1868-69
   168 Water   1871-72
   302 to 318 Water   1873
   300 W. Water   1874

Daniels, Ann (1889-98)
   439 South Broadway.   1889-98

Daniels, C. F. J. (1877-88)
   445 South Broadway   1877-82
   439 South Broadway   1882-88

Daugherty, J. W. Co. (1924-25)
   416 nec 2nd and Main   1924
   510 Wayne Ave.   1925

Davis, Andrew (1922)
   14 East Diamond Ave.   1922

Dayton Chemical Co. (1898, 1912-13)
   520 South Jackson   1898
   21 South Western Ave.   1912-13

Dayton Liniment Co. (1927-48)
   43 Illinois Ave.   1927-36
   1026 Nordale Ave.   1937-48

Dayton Medicine Co., The (1909-15)
   1st and Canal   1909
   504 South Wayne   1910-11
   32 South Jefferson   1912-13
   6 East 3rd   1914-15

Dayton Pile Cure Co. (1903-09)
   2415 East 3rd   1903-09

Dayton Pile Formula Co. (1923)
   2415 East 3rd   1923

Dayton Tanlac Agency (1917-19)
   1006 Conover Bldg.   1917-19

Dayton Viavi Co. (1899-48)***
   903 Reibold Bldg.   1899-1905

---

  *   The Brandon Medicine Co. seems to have been out of Ossco, Wisconsin.
  **   Catherine Brown was listed in 1877 as a manufacturer of "Worm Lozenges."
  *** Buckeye Medicine Co. seems to have been out of Marion, Ohio.
  **** Viavi branched out from San Francisco. Treatment for a variety of "feminine troubles."

802 U. B. Bldg.	1909-11	**Fruit-Oil-Ets Laboratories Co., The (1924)**	
401 Arcade	1912-19	616 Canby Bldg	1924
25 South Main	1921-33	**Fund, Carl (1917-18)**	
218-220 Salem Ave.	1934-48	426 East Clover	1917-18
Dickman, John P. (1903-07)		**Gebhart, M. L. (1884-85)**	
529 East Hickory	1903-07	1426 East 5th	1884-85
Dillon, Jack W. (1929)		**Globe Drug Co. (1924)**	
228 1/2 East 5th	1929	127 East 3rd	1924
Dillon, T. A. (1897-99)		**Globe Pharmaceutical Co. (1907-08, 1914-23)**	
239 East 2nd	1897-99	nec 4th and Jefferson	1907-08
Dowd, S. B. (1886-87)*		114 North St. Clair	1914-23
14 East Jones	1886-87	**Good, Martin (1888-1890)**	
13 East Springfield	1887	2415 East 5th	1888-89
Drummond's Laboratories (1932-34)		134 South Jefferson	1889-90
1913 North Main	1932	**Gore, J. I. & Co. (1916-17)***	
3122 North Main	1933	309 East 1st	1916-17
522 North Broadway	1934	**Great American Herb Co. (1900-11)****	
Duff & Shade (1908)		320 South Clay	1900-01
736 North Main	1908	30 East Marshall	1902-04
Eslinger, Katherine T. (1933-38)		506 East 5th	1905-06
401 South Main	1933-38	517 East 5th	1906-11
Eureka Medicine Co. (1913-18)**		**Grubbs, George J. (1912-13)**	
130 South Jefferson	1913-18	122 South Calm	1912-13
Evans Benjamin System Tonic Co. (1899-06)		21 West 4th	1913
331 East 3rd	1899-1905	**Hamm Remedy Co., The (1918-22)**	
302 East 3rd	1906	25 South Main	1918-22
Fant, Alfred (1908)		**Harshman, Henry R. (1890)**	
16 North Dale Ave.	1908	nwc 5th & Jefferson	1890
Fee, Fred (1917-18)		**Hart Mfg. Co. (1910-17)**	
911 East Huffman Ave.	1917-18	216 N. St. Clair	1910-17
Fegler, Arthur A. (1894-03)		**Harter, Dr. Medicine Co. (1895-1910)**	
1006 West 5th, W.S.	1894-97	nec 1st & Canal	1895-07
128 South Williams	1897-02	305 East 1st	1908-10
325 South Summit	1903	**Hasenstab, John F. (1904-18)**	
Felger Bros. & Co. (1890)		1616 East Richard	1904-05
21 North Jefferson	1890	168 South McClure	1906-07
Felix, Henry C. (1906-08)		168 South McReynolds	1907-18
609 East 2nd	1906-08	**Hauptfuehrer, August M. (1890)**	
Foley, John (1858-77)		102 South Pulaski	1890
sec 3rd and Ringold	1858-61	**Henderson Herb Co. (1915)**	
25 Terry	1862-63	53 East Sherman	1915
53 2nd	1864-65	**Hinsey, John H. (1889-06)**	
5 Clinton	1868-77	317 South Broadway	1889-01
Foose Chemical Co. (1917-24)		317 South Williams	1902-06
114 North St. Clair	1917-23	**Hinsey, Mary E. (1907-21)**	
127 East 3rd	1924	317 South Williams	1907-21

---

*   S. B. Dowd listed in 1886-87 as selling a "Catarrh Remedy."
**   Newspaper ads seem to indicate that the Eureka Medicine Company was not from Dayton.
***   J. I. Gore was an agent for the Cooper Medicine Company, jobbing out bottles of Tanlac.
****   The Great American Herb Company was out of Washington D.C.

Hirsch, Albert A. (1895-19, 1925-37)
   155 West Gorst   1895-96
   1109 South Brown   1896-98
   142 East Frank   1898-06
   114 East Frank   1907-19
   39 Huffman Ave.   1925-37
Hoefer, George J. (1929-31)
   2411 Far Hills Ave.   1929-31
Horstman, The A. Co. (1917-18)
   508 South Wayne Ave.   1917-18
Hughes, Theo. (1907-08)
   28 South Krug   1907-08
Hyre, Alfred (1897-12)
   45 East Jones   1897-12
Indian Medicine Co. (1904-06)
   303 West 3rd   1904-05
   Concord & Cincinnati   1905-06
International Proprietaries (1924-41)
   301 East 1st   1924-28
   502 East 3rd   1929-38
   1045 Third Natl. Bldg.   1939-41
Jenkins Medicine Co. (1903-06)
   2 Pocahontas Bldg.   1903-04
   226 1/2 South Ludlow   1904-05
   nwc 3rd and Terry   1905-06
Jerome, Horatio (1862-84)
   44 6th Street   1862-84
Kandoits Co., The (1902-05)
   331 East 3rd   1902-03
   329 1/2 East 3rd   1905
Kentucky Distributing Co. (1917-18)
   36 West 2nd   1917-18
Kepler, Jesse (1903)
   39 Patterson Bldg.   1903
Ketchell, Leon G. (1926)
   423 South Montgomery   1926
Ketchell, The Leon Remedy Co. (1930)
   117 Galloway   1930
Kim Chemical Co. (1914-21)
   309 East 1st   1914-21
Kintzer, Adam (1877-78)
   ss Home Ave.   1877-78
Kissinger, George (1884, 1904-07)*
   720 South Wayne   1884
   137 South Olive   1904-06
   418 West Norwood   1907

Kline, Mrs. J. J. (1896-97)
   503 South Hawthorn   1896-97
Koch, Russell W. (1922-23)
   938 North Troy   1922-23
Lang, Martin (1882-83)
   811 Brown   1882-83
Laxolet Remedy Co. (1913)
   47 Davies Bldg   1913
Leoty, Mrs. Mary (1895)
   21 East Stewart   1895
Lily Medical Co., The (1905-06)
   33 Louis Block   1905-06
Lily Remedies (1908)
   60 Davies Bldg.   1908
Littlebear, Albert (1929)
   150 Brown   1929
Livingston Remedy Co., The (1893-94)
   117 North Jefferson   1893-94
Livingston, Dr. Medicine Co. (1888)
   218 North Main   1888
Longstreet, Emma T. (1929-30)
   392 North Main   1929-30
Lovell, Stephen (1903-10)
   18 South Horton   1903-04
   251 North Alaska   1905-06
   224 North Clayton   1906-07
   164 North Clayton   1907-10
Low Brothers (1873-75)
   38 Wayne   1873-75
Low, D. B. (1871-72)
   38 Wayne   1871-72
Loyal Medicine Co. (1924-37)
   935 Cincinnati   1924-37
Lutzenberger, Charles (1910)
   swc 5th and Williams   1910
Lyndon Chemical Co, The (1923-48)
   820 Kiser   1923-48
M.I.S.T. (1895-98)**
   353 East 5th   1895-98
Mack, William (1928-29)
   816 Hart   1928
   714 Brown   1929
Ma-Ko Mfg. Co. (1915-18)
   162 North Salem   1915-18
Malt-A-Cod Laboratory Inc. (1930-36)**
   room 317, 38 East 5th   1930-36

---

* George Kissinger is listed as selling "Cathartic Worm Lozenges" in 1884.
** M.I.S.T., which stood for "Murray's Infallible System Tonic", was out of Toledo, Ohio.
*** Malt-A-Cod manufactured "Malt-A-Cod" medicine, but not in Dayton. Branch office only.

Mapello Specialty Co. (1905)
  1207 West 3rd   1905

Margo Distributing Co. (1925-43)
  209 South Ludlow   1925-36
  114 West 5th   1937-43

Marr Co., The (1927)
  207 Volkenand Avenue   1927

Marvelo Pharmaceutical Co. (1910)
  840 West 5th   1910

Mayer, August (1897-00, 1927-31)
  635 South Wayne Ave.   1897-00
  228 Plum   1927-31

McCauley, John (1884-87)
  215 South Hulbert   1884-85
  1113 East McLain   1886-87

Medco Co. (1918-21)
  114 North St. Clair   1918-21

Medical Formula Co. (1914-17)
  114 North St. Clair   1914-17

Metzger, Mary B. (1913-14)
  366 South Quitman   1913-14

Mexican Medicine Co. (1894)*
  407 East 5th   1894

Miller, C. Bert (1914-25)
  swc Washington and Cincinnati   1914-25

Miller, Edward R. (1915-32)
  156 South Irwin   1915-16
  1930 East 3rd, rear   1917-25
  419 Willowwood Drive   1926-32

Miller, Edward R. & Son (1928-31)
  419 Willowwood Drive   1928-31

Mills, Dr. John D. (1882-83)
  2nd   1882-83

Mote, Linn M. (1909-10)
  868 North Main   1909-10

National Drug Co. (1906, 1914-23)**
  524 West 3rd   1906
  532 East 1st   1914-23

National Herb Medicine Co. (1891-92)***
  420 East 5th   1891-92
  swc 5th and Stone   1892

National Laboratories, Inc. of N.Y. (1923)***
  125 East 2nd   1923

Nature's Creation (1911-12)****
  501 Conover Bldg.   1911-12

Newton, William M. (1908-10)
  30 South Garfield   1908-10

Nostriola Balm Co. (1923-39)*****
  539 Salem Ave.   1923-26
  541 Salem Ave.   1927-33
  1237 Superior Ave.   1934-39

Novita Co., The (1900-07)******
  44 Davies Bldg.   1900-01
  32 Louis Block   1902-07

Nu Method Remedy Co. (1928-29)
  207 Volkenand   1928-29

Nu-Wa Remedy Co. (1927-29)
  207 Volkenand Avenue   1927-29

Pack, Grace (1916-17)
  1016 West 3rd   1916-17

Parker, Charles H. (1923-38)
  324 East 5th   1923
  25 South Main   1924-25
  226 Irving Ave.   1926-36
  354 South Jersey   1936-38

Parker, George H. (1912-18)
  324 East 5th   1912-18

Parker, George H. & Son (1919-22)
  324 East Fifth   1919-22

Parker, H. B. (1932)
  208 South Ludlow   1932

Parson Pharmacal Co., The (1919-20)
  11 North St. Mary's   1919-20

Pew, Albert A. Co. (1907-08)
  346 East Jones   1907-08

Portage Chemical Co., The (1903)
  537 East 1st   1903

Potter, Ira A. & Co. (1891-13)
  8 1/2 South Brown   1891-02
  634 South Wayne Ave.   1903-05
  2032 East 3rd   1906-13

Prescription Products Co. (1908-15)
  203 South Summit   1908-09
  314 South College   1910-15

Pretzinger Catarrh Balm Co. (1905-22)
  41 East 3rd   1905-12

---

*   The Mexican Medicine Co. made "Ko-Ds - The Great Mexican Blood Tonic", but not in Dayton.
**   The National Drug Co. was out of Washington, D.C.
***   National Herb Medicine Co. was out of Detroit, Michigan.
****   National Laboratories, Inc. of N.Y. was out of New York.
***** Nature's Cure had branch offices across the U.S. Sold as a cure for nearly every disease.
****** Nostriola Balm Co., of Wheeling, West Virginia, opened branch here to sell "Mus-Tur-Pep."
******* The Novita Company was out of Lima, Ohio.

33 East 3rd	1913-22	**Schoene, Dr. J. Z. (1889)**	
Pretzinger, R. & Bro. (1896-04)		East Helena Street	1889
41 East 3rd	1896-04	**Schuder, Christian L. (1904-05)**	
Private Formula Co. (1893-03)		1419 West Germantown	1904-05
317 North Taylor	1893-98	**Scott & Richardson (1898)**	
40 South Main	1900-01	nec Shank & Toledo	1898
207 East 2nd	1902-03	**Scott, Andrew J. (1893-00)**	
905 West 3rd	1903	61 South Terry	1893-00
Psoric Institute (1932-44)		**Sellman, William (1894-97, 1904-16)**	
room 549, 38 East 5th	1932-33	64 South Eagle	1894-97
1016 Superior Ave.	1934-44	26 East Mumma Ave.	1904-16
Raines, John W. (1907-13)		**Shade Medicine Co. (1927-38)**	
512 East 1st	1907-09	1125 North Main, rear	1927-32
744 South Main	1910-11	1838 North Main	1933
35 South Tecumseh	1912-13	**Shade, George W. & Co. (1909-25)**	
Rall, Joseph T. (1881-83, 1886-87, 1893-94)		823 North Main	1909-12
36 East 4th	1881-82	1125 North Main, rear	1913-25
306 Wayne Ave.	1882-83	**Sheets & Eby (1858-59)**	
118 South Terry	1886-87	sec 1st and Jefferson	1858-59
1219 East 3rd	1893-94	**Sheets, Andrew (1860-61)**	
Rall, Joseph T. & Son (1884-85)		sec 1st and Jefferson	1860-61
308 South Wayne	1884-85	**Shroyer, Andrew (1894-97)**	
Ramona Herb Co. (1917-21)		25 East Jones	1894-95
208 South Ludlow	1917-18	swc 3rd & Home Ave.	1895-96
111 South Jefferson	1918-21	23 West 5th	1896-97
Rarich, Henry J. (1874-77)		**Shroyer, Andrew J. (1900-02)**	
46 Herrman	1874-77	Findlay near Valley	1900-02
Redfern Medicine Co. (1927-33)		**Sisson Drug Co. (1933-36)***	
1048 Redfern Avenue	1927-33	1231 U B Bldg.	1933-36
Redwood Medicine Co. (1926-38)		**Smith, Jesse C. (1911-14)**	
1125 North Main, rear	1926	1151 West 3rd	1911-12
945 U. B. Bldg.	1927-30	1016 West 3rd	1913-14
1135 U. B. Bldg.	1931-38	**Smith, S. N. & Co. (1875-96)**	
Rowling, Amza W. (1887-88)		alley btwn 2nd & 3rd	1875-83
106 South King, W.S.	1887-88	1308 West 3rd, W.S.	1884-96
Royal Remedy & Extract Co., The (1880-97)		**Smith, Walter (1894)**	
453 East 5th	1880	1641 East 5th	1894
14 West 2nd	1881-85	**Smyrna Bitters Co. (1909-14)**	
14 West 2nd	1884-85	506 South Wayne Ave.	1909-12
21 East 2nd	1886-97	39 East Jones	1913-14
Sal-Phenine Laboratories Inc. (1930-38)		**Smyrna Products Co., The (1915)**	
208 South Ludlow	1930-38	1902 East 5th	1915
Sanitos Medical Co. (1902)		**Spengler's Rheumatic Remedy (1897-98)**	
922 South Wayne	1902	nec 2nd & Webster	1897-98
Sargon Laboratories Inc. (1930-34)		**Spoon, Melvin E. (1927)**	
301 East 1st	1930-34	2759 Home Ave.	1927
Schmoll Medicine Co. (1898-00)		**Swartz, David H. (1903)**	
nwc 5th and Huffman	1898-00	36 West Washington	1903

* Sisson Drug Company was out of Columbus, Ohio.
** The Smyrna Bitters Co. manufactured a "stomach bitters" which they claimed "Prolongs Life."

T & A Chemical Co. (1909-13)
   45 Davies Bldg.   1909-10
   21 Callahan Bldg.   1911
   39 West McPherson   1912-13
Texas Post Oak Co. (1906)
   506 East 2nd   1906
Thill & Bacher (1916-17)
   531 South Steele Ave.   1916-17
Tona Vita Medicine Co. (1914-17)
   125 South Ludlow   1914-17
Treatine Laboratories Inc. (1933)
   502 Wayne Avenue   1933
Tressler, Harry A. (1928)
   2411 Far Hills Ave.   1928
United States Manufacturing Co. (1884-86)
   352 South Main   1884-85
   422 East 5th   1886
Victory Remedy Co, The (1905-07)
   203 South Summit, rear   1905-07
Vi-Dermis Co, The (1907-13)
   swc 3rd and Jefferson   1907-13
Vin Hepatica Co. (1915-17)
   16 South St. Clair   1915
   24 North Jefferson   1916-17
Vinco Herb Co., The (1921-41)
   549 North Salem Ave.   1921-24
   541 Salem Ave.   1925-33
   1237 Superior Ave.   1934-41
Vinos Products Co., The (1926)
   515 East Herman Ave.   1926
Vionna Co. The (1911)
   nec 1st and Canal   1911
Wain, Thomas (1893)
   1311 East 3rd   1893
Waltz, John A. (1898)
   434 East Clover   1898
Weis Bros. Medicine Co., The (1911-12)
   415 East 5th   1911-12
Weis, The Dr. H. F. Medicine Co. (1876-23)
   706 South Wayne Ave.   1876-21
   605 East 5th   1922-23
Wells Mfg. Co. (1933)
   525 South Williams   1933
West Side Cut Rate Medicine Store (1906-07)
   1151 West 3rd   1906-07
White, Channing (1881)
   216 North Main   1881
Wietzel Drug Co. (1909-25)
   400 East 5th   1909-25
Willson, James (1904)
   338 South Srague   1904

Wood, Benjamin M. (1862-63)
   234 5th Street   1862-63
Workman, Percy W. (1923-24)
   35 Madison   1923-24
Wright, I. H. (1919-25)
   911 East Huffman Ave.   1919-25
Yarwood, Albert W. (1917-18)
   1016 West 3rd   1917-18
Younce, Davis (1874-78)
   923 W. 3rd, W.S.   1874
   swc Brown and Shartel   1875-77
   13 Washington   1877-78
Young, Lewis R. (1902-14)
   121 West Leroy   1902-07
   64 West Weller   1908-09
   1419 West Germantown   1909-12
   608 South Summit   1913-14
Younge, James E. (1924-25)
   nec 2nd and Main   1924
   510 Wayne Avenue   1925
Zellars, Carrie (1914-15)
   407 North Broadway   1914-15
Zo-Ro-Lo of Dayton   (1932-37)
   1601 U. B. Bldg.   1932-35
   9 Davies Bldg.   1936
   25 Davies Bldg.   1937
Zuebelen Medicine Co. (1927-28)
   125 Salem Avenue   1927-28

Index & Photo Credits

This index does not repeat the list in the section, "Patent Medicine Sellers in Dayton 1850-1933".

A.B.C. Products, 61
Adams, Samuel Hopkins, 33, 79-82, 89
Ainsworth, Claire, 75-76
American Drug Company, The, 49-50
American Medical Association, 89
Anderson, Hardman, 57
Approved Formula Company, The, 47
Arras, Ann, 56
Arras, Nicholas, 56
Arras's Celebrated Remedies, 56
Baker, Lewis, 68-69
Beard, Frances, 70
Beard, Oliver P., 70
Bell, E. C., 32
Blackburn Products Company, 64-69, 75, 77
Blackburn, Ira Robert, 64-67, 75
Blackburn's Balmwort Tablets, 65
Blackburn's Cadomene Tablets, 72
Blackburn's CascaRoyal Pills, 64-65
Blackburn's Castor-Oil Pills, 64
Blackburn's Compound Fluid Balmwort, 65
Blackburn's Essence of Mentho-Laxene, 67
Blackburn's Gloriol Tonique Astringent, 75
Blackburn's Hypo-Nuclane, 75
Blackburn's Medicated Venosol, 77
Blackburn's Mentho-Laxene salve, 66
Blackburn's Phythyrin Tablets, 77
Blackburn's Quinoxide Tablets, 75
Blackburn's Rose-Kayloin, 75
Blackburn's Sulpherb Tablets, 66
Blackburn's Su-Thol Tablets, 66, 72
Blackburn's Triopeptine Tablets, 68
Blackburn's Vilane Powder, 65
Bloch, Ivan, 73
Blodgett, William, 11
Boston Cough Balm, 57
Botanic Lung Syrup, 48
Botanic Remedy Company, 48
Bowanee Medicine Company, 13
Buckeye Bottle Works, 38
Burge-Layton Company, 50
Burgess, Mr., 11-12
Burgess, Mrs. 12
C. I. Hood Company, 27
Carter Medicine Company, 55
Carter's Little Liver Pills, 55
CascaRoyal Pills, 64-65
Cheney, F. J., 84
Chiles, J. W., 43

Concentrated Oil of Pine, 56
Connecticut Agricultural Experiment Station, 47, 75
Continental Ointment, 63
Continental Specialty Company, 63
Conway, Edward, 7
Cooper Medicine Company, 12, 29-34, 48
Cooper, G. H., 29
Cooper, James, 29
Cooper, Jesse, 29, 32
Cooper, Joseph A., 32-33
Cooper, Lee T., 29-36
Cooper, Mary, 29
Cooper, W. R., 50
Cooper, William R., 29, 50
Cooper's New Discovery, 29, 31, 33, 35
Cooper's Quick Relief, 30, 33
Courcey, M. D., 78
Crook, James, 20
Crook, Oliver 20-23, 44-45
Daniels, Ann, 14
Daniels, C. F. J., 14
Davisson, Oscar F., 27
Dayton Advertising Club, 67
Dayton Board of Health, 9
Dayton Board of Trade, 27
Dayton Brewry Company, 38
Dayton Medicine Company, 35
Detrick, Daniel, 8
Dietary Supplement Health and Education Act, 90
Dingell, John D., 90
Dr. Baird's Remedy, 70
Dr. Crook's Benzoin Elixir, 22, 44
Dr. Crook's Citron Balsam, 22
Dr. Crook's Compound Syrup of Poke Root, 45
Dr. Crook's S-PH-L-S, 22, 74
Dr. Crook's Vegetable Extract, 22, 44
Dr. Crook's Wine of Tar, 21-23, 44, 87
Dr. DuChoine's Female Regulating Pills, 71
Dr. DuChoine's Nerve Pills, 72
Dr. E. Conway's Liniment, 7
Dr. Evan's Imperial Pain Cure, 15
Dr. H. F. Weis Medicine Company, 40
Dr. H. F. Weis' Tape Worm Remedy, 35
Dr. Harter & Company, 25
Dr. Harter Medicine Company, 24-27, 35, 55, 71, 73, 84-86, 88
Dr. Harter's Elixir of Wild Cherry, 24, 27
Dr. Harter's Fever, Ague & Neuralgia Specific, 25, 27
Dr. Harter's German Vermifuge Candy, 35

Dr. Harter's Iron Tonic, 27-28
Dr. Harter's Liniment, 27
Dr. Harter's Little Liver Pills, 27, 55
Dr. Harter's Lung Balm, 27
Dr. Harter's Magic Tonic, 28
Dr. Harter's Wild Cherry Bitters, 27
Dr. J. Kramer's Eye Salve, 59
Dr. Livingston Medicine Company, 14
Dr. Livingston's Positive Cure for Catarrh, 14
Dr. Oliver Crook & Co., 87
Dr. Proctor's Wine of Tar, 21
Dr. Rose's Strong Wine of Life, 20
Dr. Weis' Worm Salve, 35
Durham-Humphrey Act, 90
Eichelberger, Daniel H., 23
Epidemic of 1811 in Dayton, 9
Evans, M., 15
F. Beard Company, 70
First Presbyterian Church, 87
Foley, Abigail, 52
Foley, John, 51-52
Food and Drug Administration, 46, 90
Foose, A. P., 56, 77
Foote, John T., 33
G. W. Shade & Company, 54
Garst, M., 9
Gebhart, Edgar S., 53
Geiger, Alburtus, 20, 23
Geiger, George H., 17-18
German Vermifuge Candy, 35
Globe Pharmaceutical Company, 56, 77
Gold Cure, 17
Great American Fraud, The, 33, 89
Great American Herb Company, 54
Great Dropsy Remedy, 40-41
Great East Indian Tonic, 16
Great Indian Asthma and Hay Fever Remedy, 54
Great Nova Scotia Pain Killer, 14
Green, Benjamin, 13
Green, Harry, 13
Guard on the Rhine, 40
Gump, Andrew, 23
Gump, William E., 23
Haines, Job, 9, 11
Hall's Catarrh Cure, 84
Harter, Milton G., 24-25
Harter, Samuel K., 25, 27
Hauer Music Company, 38
Hayner Distilling Company, 27
Hayner, William M., 25, 27
Health and Beauty, booklet, 69
Hefferline, John W., 78
Hinsey, John H., 16
Hinsey, Mary, 16
Hirsch, Albert A., 46, 59
Hirsch's Ambition Tablets, 59
Hirsch's Kidney, Liver and Bladder Regulator, ad 46

Hirsch's Sarsaparilla, 46
Hollister, Howard, 33
Houser, H. C., 15
How to be Beautiful, newspaper column, 75
Hunter, W. W., 14
Indian Herb Tablets, 54
Indian Medicine Company, 54
Indianapolis, Indiana, 32
International Proprietaries, Inc., 34, 48
J. Foley's Indian Botanic Balsam, 51-52
Johnson, J. N., 54
Josse, Peter, 78
Journal of the American Medical Association, 33, 65, 70, 89
Ka-Vita, 35
K-D Kidney Tablets, 60
Kefauver-Harris Amendment, 90
Ki-A-Wah, 54
Kidder, Walter S., 25, 27
Kirves, Bruno, 17
Kirves, Emma, 17
Kirves, Mary, 17
Koogler, Dr., 20
Krehbiel, Andrew J., 8
Krehbiel, Louisa A., 8
Kurokol, 12
Lannon, Augusta, 20
Leslie Company, 75
Lexington, Kentucky, 31, 33
Live & Let Live Drug Store, 80
Livingston, E. B., 14
Louisville, Kentucky, 70
Low Brothers, 62
Low, Charles M., 62
Low, David B., 62
Low's Electric Liniment, 62
McCabe's Market, ad, 35
Middletown, Ohio, 54
Miller, Augustus, 13
Miller, John W., 65
Miller, William, 13
Montgomery County Medical Society, 10, 20, 23
Morrissey, Ed, 32
Nautch Girl, The, 87
Neave, J. L., 51
New Haven Department of Health, 47
Newman, David S., 9
North American Indian Doctor, The, book, 51
Nostrums and Quackery, book, 33-34, 89
O'Donnell, D. J., 49
Oland, Conrad G., 38
Park Presbyterian Church, 23
Park, John D., 23
Parker, Charles, 54
Parker, George H., 54
Parker's K. & P. Pink Herb Tablets, 54
Pepgen Laxative, 49-50

Pepgen Liniment, 49-50
Pepgen, tonic, 6, 49-50
Perkins, Ellen E., 73
Pilkington, William E., 56, 77
Polan, Floyd, 32
Potter, Ira A., 58
Potter's Plasters, 58
Presbyterian Cookbook, 87
Prescription Products Company, 75
Pretzinger Bros., 42
Pretzinger, Albert, 42
Pretzinger, Herman, 42
Pretzinger, Rudolph, 42
Pretzinger's Catarrh Balm, 42
Pretzinger's Nasal Balm, 42
Pruden, David, 38
Pure Food and Drugs Act, 33, 49, 54, 56, 64, 90
R. & R. Sign Company, 54
Ramona Herb Company, 46
Ra-Mo-Na Herbs Tablets, 46
red letter clause, 84
Redfern Medicine Company, 53
Redfern, Robert, 53
Redfern's Indian Tonic, 53
Redwood Medicine Company, 60-61
Redwood's Liniment, 61
Revenue Act of 1862, 23
Rice, Elwood E., 54
Rose, James S., 18-20
Rouzer, William H., 23
Royal Remedy and Extract Company, 57
Royal Remedy Company, 57
Rumex Medicine Company, 15
Rumex, 15
S. N. Smith & Co., 23, 59
Sachs & Pruden Drug Store, 38
Sach's Lithia Water, 38
Sachs, Edward, 38
Sachs-Pruden Ale Company, 38
Sachs-Pruden's A-T-8 Agaric, 38-39, 88
Saline Lemonade, 38
Sartoin Skin Food, 77
Scheigert, Louis, 32
Shade Medicine, 54

Sherley Amendment, 90
Skip, 61
Smith, S. N., 23
Smith, Silas H., 9
Souder's Boston Cough Balm, 57
Souders, Irvin C., 57
Spengler, John G., 36
Spengler's Drug Store, 36
Spengler's Rheumatic Remedy, 36
St. Bonifacius Gentian Flower Tonic, 43
St. Bonifacius Liver Pill, 43
St. Bonifacius Oak Oil, 43
St. Bonifacius Remedy Company, 43
St. Bonifacius Rose Ointment, 43
St. Bonifacius Toothache Drops, 43
St. Bonifacius Wild Cherry Cough Cure, 43
Sweetman, J. E. (Mrs.), 72
Tanlac Vegetable Pills, 48
Tanlac, 33-34, 48, 79-83, 85
The Doctor's Advice, newspaper column, 68
Tona Vita, 47
Trimbach, Joseph, 33
Tripler, Mr., 80
Tripler, V. W. (Mrs.), 79-81
Troy, Ohio, 24-25, 27
Unparalleled Recipes, 8
van Wassenaur, Nicholaes, 51
Victory Remedy Company, 64
Weis, Henry F., 40-41
Wentworth, L., 35
West Side Civic Association, 67
West Uhrich, Ohio, 32
Wick, Fred, 83
Wietzel Drug Store, 37
Wietzel, Christopher J., 37
Wietzel's Stomach and Bowel Tonic, 37
Williams, H. J., 54
Williamson, Homer, 32
Willis, G. F., 33, 80-81
Winders, Frank, 32
Wine of Tar Picture Alphabet, booklet, 21
Wingert, Alfred Lenahan, 82
Winters, B. H., 27
Zelax Indian Herb Tablets, 37

Photo Credits

James D. Julia, Inc., Auctioners - Three-panel Tanlac display, cover. **Frank Miller** - Pepgen display, 6, Pepgen Liniment bottle, 50. **Dayton Metro Library** - cure book, 8, Medical Society fee bill, 10, Wine of Tar picture book, 21-22, Royal Remedy trade card, 57. **John Wolf** - Dr. Evan's Imperial Pain Cure bottle, 15, Crook's Vegetable Syphilitic Remedy bottle, 74. **Friends of Hayner for the items located in the Hayner Distillery Exhibition, Troy-Hayner Cultural Center, Troy, OH** - Dr. Harter's Wild Cherry bottle, 24, Dr. Harter's Fever & Ague bottle, 25, Dr. Harter's Iron Tonic Compound box, 28, Harter's Little Liver Pills bottles, 55. **Dana Wiehl** - Cooper's Quick Relief box, 30. **Marianne Foster** - St. Bonifacus trade card, 43. **John McCutcheon** - Syrup of Poke Root bottle, 45. **John Bartley** - Tona Vita bottle, 47. **Scott & Carol Davis** - Pepgen box and bottle, 49. **Mike Smith** - J. Foley's Indian Botanic Balsam bottles, 52. **Nick Blackburn** - Casca Royal Pills tin, 64, Essence of Mentho-Laexene bottle and box, 67. **All other items either owned by author or by donors who wish to remain anonymous.**

www.ingramcontent.com/pod-product-compliance
Lightning Source LLC
Chambersburg PA
CBHW050729180526
45159CB00003B/1168